Elixir of Eudaimonia

"Unveiling the Illusion of Perfection"

By

DR FAITH STONES

Table of Contents

Introduction

In the radiant world of Eudaimonia, where every dawn paints the sky with hues of serenity and every smile is genuine, the pursuit of perfection is an art form. The heartbeats of its citizens resonate with the rhythm of health, and laughter flows like a fragrant breeze through its streets. But amid the harmonious melody of life, there exists an undertone—a whisper of curiosity that tugs at the corners of reality, inviting one young soul to embark on a journey that will forever transform the symphony of Eudaimonia.

Meet Ava, a curious spirit with eyes that harbor unspoken questions and a heart that beats to the rhythm of a world not yet known. Within the holographic displays that paint her city with the colors of unity, Ava glimpses fleeting shadows— glimmers of doubt that hint at a truth beyond the facade. It is through a chance encounter with Emma, an enigmatic figure from a realm beyond Eudaimonia's borders, that Ava's path takes a daring turn.

As they walk together beneath the stars, Emma unfolds tales of lands where the boundaries of health and happiness have yielded to the enigma of authenticity. Her words are like stardust, casting sparks of curiosity into the vast canvas of Ava's imagination. Within her, a fire awakens—an ember of realization that the world she knows may be but a reflection of the truth that waits to be unveiled.

Bound by courage and fueled by curiosity, Ava embarks on a journey that will lead her beyond the veil of perfection and into the heart of Eudaimonia's secrets. In the company of rebels and thinkers, skeptics and dreamers, she will navigate the labyrinth of illusion, daring to question the very elixir that sustains her world. As the lines between harmony and authenticity blur, Ava's footsteps echo with the promise of change, and the symphony of Eudaimonia finds itself on the precipice of transformation.

"Elixir of Eudaimonia" is a tale of discovery and revelation, where the pursuit of truth ignites a flame that transcends the confines of perfection. Join Ava on a journey that will not only challenge the foundation of her society but also inspire readers to contemplate the delicate balance between utopia and reality, between the elixirs we seek and the authenticity we yearn for.

Chapter 1:

Perfect Utopia

The sun painted the sky with hues of pink and gold as Ava emerged from her apartment. The seamless glass door slid open with a soft whisper, revealing a world that seemed to have been meticulously designed by an artist with an obsession for perfection. Eudaimonia's streets were clean and orderly, a symphony of white and silver against the backdrop of a cloudless azure sky. Each building stood as a testament to architectural mastery, blending seamlessly with the surrounding natural beauty.

Ava's footsteps echoed in rhythm with her heartbeat as she made her way through the city's pedestrian paths. The air carried a hint of floral fragrance, a result of the genetically engineered flowers that adorned every corner. A gentle breeze stirred her hair, and Ava's gaze lifted to the horizon, where the sun bathed everything in a warm, inviting glow.

Smiles greeted her at every turn, friends and acquaintances acknowledging her with a nod or a wave. Conversations flowed like a gentle stream, and laughter harmonized with the gentle hum of technology. Yet, beneath the surface of her perfect interactions, Ava carried a weight that no amount of technology could alleviate. She was a mosaic of contradictions—a physical embodiment of health, yet an emotional realm dominated by restlessness.

Amid the sea of radiant faces, Ava often found herself lost in thought, questioning the authenticity of their interactions. Did they truly care, or were these exchanges merely the expected choreography of Eudaimonia's social dance? Beneath the surface, her eyes held a faint trace of longing, a reflection of a yearning for something more profound.

As Ava walked, she couldn't help but notice the ever-present screens that adorned buildings and public spaces. Holographic projections displayed the latest medical advancements, narrating a saga of triumphs over diseases that once plagued humanity.

The technology of Eudaimonia was nothing short of miraculous, but Ava couldn't shake off the nagging thought that something essential had been lost in the pursuit of perfection.

Ava's path eventually led her to the heart of the city—a sprawling plaza dominated by a mesmerizing fountain. Water danced in intricate patterns, catching the sunlight and scattering it into dazzling fragments. People gathered around, their laughter a cheerful melody that harmonized with the fountain's song. The screens embedded in the ground displayed scrolling news, celebrating another year without a single instance of illness.

Ava stood on the periphery of the crowd, a participant yet an observer. Applause erupted as the news concluded, voices overlapping in a chorus of elation. She smiled, her lips curving in sync with societal expectations, yet her thoughts were far away. Was perfect health truly the pinnacle of existence, or was there more to life than the absence of physical maladies?

As the sun dipped below the horizon, bathing the plaza in hues of gold and tangerine, Ava felt an inexplicable pull towards a nearby park. The lush greenery unfolded before her like a living canvas. Trees, meticulously pruned, created an atmosphere of tranquility, while technologically enhanced birdsong filled the air with a melody that was both enchanting and eerie in its precision.

She wandered along a cobblestone path, each step accompanied by the soft crunch of gravel. The beauty was undeniable, yet a sense of unease gnawed at her. The air was pure, the environment untouched by toxins, yet the world she inhabited felt too controlled, too sterile. It was as if the relentless pursuit of perfection had distilled life into an almost monochromatic existence.

Ava paused at the edge of the park, her gaze fixed on the horizon where the first stars emerged, blinking like distant diamonds. In this moment of quiet contemplation, a memory surged to the forefront of her mind—a memory of an old book, ancient by Eudaimonia's standards, tucked away in a forgotten corner of the city's vast archives.

The book was a relic from a time when humanity battled against the very imperfections that

Eudaimonia had eradicated. It spoke of struggles, of victories not just over illness but over the human spirit's capacity to overcome adversity. In its pages, Ava had glimpsed a world unburdened by physical perfection yet enriched by the human experience in all its shades.

With a wistful smile, Ava allowed herself to be enveloped by the park's serene embrace. In this pocket of nature, her thoughts flowed freely, and a spark of curiosity ignited within her. What if there was more to life than the pursuit of physical well-being? What if true happiness lay in embracing the entirety of the human experience, both its triumphs and its tribulations?

As the stars overhead multiplied in number, Ava made a silent promise to herself. She would uncover the truths hidden beneath Eudaimonia's gleaming facade, even if it meant challenging the very foundations of the perfect utopia.

Absolutely, here's a detailed expansion of Chapter 2: "The Facade of Happiness," with around 900 words. This chapter delves deeper into Ava's daily life and interactions, revealing her growing sense of discontent despite the outward appearance of happiness. Remember, you can add more descriptions, thoughts, and dialogue to further enhance the chapter:

Chapter 2:

The Facade of Happiness

The next morning, Ava's apartment was bathed in soft, simulated sunlight as she rose from her meticulously designed sleep pod. The pod had monitored her vitals throughout the night, adjusting temperature and lighting to ensure optimal rest. As she stretched, a holographic screen on the wall displayed her health metrics: heart rate, blood pressure, and more—all perfectly within the desired ranges.

As she dressed in clothing that seemed to meld with her body's contours, Ava's gaze lingered on her reflection. Every feature was flawlessly symmetrical, her skin seemingly untouched by the passage of time. But the emptiness she'd felt for months was as present as ever. She touched the mirror's surface, her fingertips tracing a whisper-thin crack in the glass—a crack that had appeared mysteriously, defying the otherwise pristine perfection of her surroundings.

Breakfast was an assembly of nutrient-rich dishes, each portion calibrated to provide her body with precisely what it needed. Ava ate alone, the holographic news projected onto the table's surface. The headlines spoke of new medical achievements, life expectancies extending ever further. But as she scanned the articles, her thoughts drifted to Professor Caine's words about the value of a life rich in experiences.

Work was a flurry of activity as Ava navigated her role as a communication specialist, interacting with holographic interfaces and attending virtual meetings with colleagues. Conversations flowed effortlessly, colleagues expressing genuine pleasure at her company. Yet, even in these exchanges, Ava sensed a shallowness—a reluctance to delve into topics beyond the superficial.

Lunchtime found her in a communal eating area, surrounded by people engrossed in conversations that rarely ventured beyond the realms of health and fitness. As Ava ate her nutrient-rich salad, she listened to the buzz around her. "My workout regimen just got upgraded. Can't wait to see the results." "I heard they're introducing a new longevity treatment next month." The words were a chorus of contentment, yet Ava couldn't shake the feeling that something fundamental was missing.

After work, Ava joined friends at an art exhibit showcasing holographic sculptures that seemed to dance with light and color. She exchanged pleasantries, admired the art, and engaged in discussions about the aesthetic value of the pieces. But beneath the facade of her smile, a yearning lingered—a yearning for conversations that delved beyond aesthetics, that explored the human experience in all its complexity.

The evening air was crisp as Ava strolled through Eudaimonia's streets, heading towards a recreational area where groups of people engaged in physical activities. Some jogged along the illuminated paths, their strides effortless and graceful. Others practiced yoga or engaged in holographically simulated sports. Ava stood by, observing, her gaze drifting over the faces that radiated vitality.

As darkness descended, Ava found herself beneath the city's shimmering skyline. She leaned against a railing, gazing out at the expanse of perfection that lay before her. The stars above seemed brighter than ever, a reminder of the universe's vastness—a contrast to the microcosm of controlled beauty that she inhabited.

Amidst the harmonious blend of technological achievements and architectural brilliance, Ava's heart felt a profound isolation. The very attributes that made Eudaimonia a utopia seemed to strip away the depth of human connection—the vulnerability, the shared struggles, the raw authenticity that defined the human experience.

As she turned to leave, Ava's gaze fell upon a holographic screen that displayed a quote by an ancient philosopher: "The unexamined life is not worth living." The words lingered in the air, a whisper of truth amid the gleaming facade. With a newfound determination, Ava walked away, her steps echoing with a resolve to uncover the layers of her existence that lay beyond the surface.

Chapter 3:

Forbidden Knowledge

In the heart of Eudaimonia's sprawling library, Ava's fingers danced over the smooth surfaces of holographic interfaces, each touch a gateway to endless information. Yet, her gaze was fixed on one particular terminal—the one that held records of a bygone era, a time before perfect health was a birthright.

With a mixture of anticipation and trepidation, Ava accessed the section of the archives that contained the ancient texts. Her heart raced as she scrolled through titles, feeling like an explorer unearthing forgotten artifacts. And then she saw it—a title that seemed to call out to her amidst the sea of forgotten wisdom.

The book was encased in an ornate holographic shell, its appearance almost out of place in Eudaimonia's sleek environment. With a deep breath, Ava touched the shell, and it unfolded, revealing pages that resembled parchment, each illuminated by a soft, ethereal light. She was holding a relic from a past where physical perfection was an aspiration, not an expectation.

As Ava read the words, her heart quickened, and her mind was transported to a world where health was a battle, not a given. The book spoke of something called "eudaimonia," a Greek word that suggested a state of true well-being, a life rich in purpose and meaning. The text described how ancient philosophers had explored the interplay between physical health, mental well-being, and the pursuit of a life worth living.

The concept fascinated Ava. She found herself drawn into the words as if they were a lifeline to a realm she had yet to explore—a realm that seemed to resonate with the emptiness she felt despite her perfect health. The more she read, the more she became entranced by the idea that well-being was more than the absence of illness—it was a tapestry woven from experiences, relationships, and personal growth.

Ava lost track of time as she immersed herself in the ancient wisdom. It was a world of contrasts: the Eudaimonia she lived in was a monument to human achievements in health, while the world of the past celebrated the intricate dance of the human spirit. She realized that the pursuit of eudaimonia was not about escaping imperfections; it was about embracing them as integral threads in the fabric of a meaningful existence.

As the words danced before her eyes, Ava was interrupted by a voice—a voice that seemed to belong to another era. "Ah, I see you've found the book."

Startled, Ava looked up to see an older man standing before her, his eyes crinkling with a warm smile. His appearance was in stark contrast to the pristine citizens of Eudaimonia; his hair was tinged with silver, his face etched with lines that told stories of a life fully lived.

"I apologize if I startled you," the man continued, extending a hand. "I'm Professor Caine."

Ava hesitated, her fingers tightening around the book. "I'm Ava," she replied cautiously, her eyes narrowing as she studied him. His presence felt like a ripple in the carefully orchestrated serenity of Eudaimonia.

Professor Caine's gaze met hers with an understanding that seemed to stretch beyond the surface. "You're curious about the book," he said, his voice a blend of reassurance and intrigue.

Ava nodded, her heart pounding as she wondered how much he knew about her fascination with the ancient text.

"I've spent a lifetime exploring the forgotten depths of human wisdom," Professor Caine said, his voice tinged with a hint of nostalgia. "Eudaimonia is a marvel of achievement, but it's essential to remember that the pursuit of perfection can sometimes obscure the true essence of well-being."

Ava's curiosity mingled with caution. How much could she trust this man? But the pull of his words was undeniable—the echo of a sentiment she had begun to embrace.

"I believe," Professor Caine continued, "that there's more to well-being than meets the eye. The pursuit of eudaimonia encompasses not just physical health, but the richness of experiences, relationships, and personal growth. It's a journey that leads to a life truly worth living."

Ava looked down at the ancient book in her hands, its pages glowing with ancient wisdom. She felt a stirring within her—a resonance with the idea that there was more to her existence than the surface-level interactions of Eudaimonia.

With a mixture of determination and vulnerability, Ava met Professor Caine's gaze. "Tell me more," she said, her voice a whispered invitation to dive deeper into the world he seemed to embody—a world that held the promise of answers to the questions that had been haunting her.

Chapter 4:

Eudaimonia's Origin

In the heart of Eudaimonia's sprawling library, Professor Caine guided Ava through the dimly lit aisles, each step echoing with anticipation. The ancient texts, bound in faded leather and inscribed with the knowledge of generations past, were a testament to a world that had existed before perfect health became the ultimate goal. Ava's fingers brushed against the timeworn spines, feeling a connection to a time she had only heard about in whispers.

Settling into a comfortable alcove, Ava looked at Professor Caine with eager eyes. His presence radiated a sense of wisdom, as if he were a living bridge to the past.

"Long before Eudaimonia," Professor Caine began, his voice a rich tapestry of experiences, "humanity grappled with the fragile nature of life. Disease, suffering, and mortality were the constants that shaped existence. But within the hearts of some individuals, a dream was born—a dream of a world where these afflictions were mere memories."

Ava leaned in, her imagination ignited by the prospect of a world vastly different from her own.

"The founders of Eudaimonia," Professor Caine continued, his eyes reflecting the flicker of memory, "were visionaries who saw a future beyond the limitations of the past. They believed that science could transform society, that technology could rewrite the script of human existence."

Ava's gaze drifted to the holographic images projected around them, depicting the founders in a state of fervent innovation, their hands sketching blueprints and equations on transparent screens.

"The journey to Eudaimonia was a monumental endeavor," Professor Caine explained. "The founders harnessed the power of genetic engineering, nanotechnology, and AI to create a society where perfect health was no longer an aspiration—it was the norm."

As images of laboratories and bustling research facilities filled the air, Ava marveled at the collective determination that had given birth to her utopian world.

"Yet," Professor Caine's tone grew somber, "achieving such a society came at a price—a price often overlooked in the celebration of progress. The very pursuit of perfect health required sacrifices that altered the essence of humanity."

Ava's brows furrowed as she considered the implications. "What kind of sacrifices?"

"To eliminate illness and suffering," Professor Caine replied, "the founders had to redefine the boundaries of what it meant to be human. They enhanced genetic traits, eradicated vulnerabilities, and developed regenerative technologies that extended life spans indefinitely."

Images of medical marvels unfolded before them, showcasing individuals undergoing treatments that seemed both awe-inspiring and unsettling.

"However," Professor Caine continued, "these advancements demanded a trade-off. To achieve perfect health, emotions had to be regulated. Joy and sorrow, love and heartache—they were all dampened, muted, in an effort to create a society where emotional turmoil was no longer a concern."

Ava's heart ached at the thought of a world devoid of the emotional spectrum that made humanity so beautifully complex.

"Eudaimonia's founders believed they were shaping a paradise," Professor Caine said, "a world where suffering had been vanquished. But in their pursuit of perfection, they inadvertently traded authenticity for surface-level interactions, emotional depth for sanitized contentment."

Images of Eudaimonia's citizens engaged in activities that seemed more like choreographed rituals than genuine expressions of emotion played across the holographic screens.

"Over time," Professor Caine continued, "the citizens of Eudaimonia began to equate well-being solely with the absence of physical maladies. The importance of emotional connection and personal growth faded into the background, overshadowed by the pursuit of physical perfection."

Ava's thoughts whirled as she grasped the enormity of the story. Eudaimonia's birth was not merely a triumph of science—it was a complex interplay of choices and consequences.

"Eudaimonia's history," Professor Caine concluded, "is a testament to human ingenuity and the unintended repercussions of progress. As you've seen, perfection came at the cost of embracing the entirety of the human experience—the vulnerabilities, the imperfections, and the intricate tapestry that defines us."

Silence enveloped the alcove as Ava processed the weight of the story. Eudaimonia was built on choices—choices that had forever altered the course of human evolution. It was a society born of aspirations, driven by a desire to banish suffering, yet one that had sacrificed something irreplaceable in the process.

"I believe," Professor Caine's gaze met Ava's, "that rekindling the essence of eudaimonia—the holistic well-being that encompasses all facets of human life—is the key to rediscovering the depth of existence."

Ava nodded, her mind racing with the newfound understanding. The journey ahead was uncertain, but the truths she had uncovered—the truths that lay buried in the past—beckoned her to venture beyond the confines of surface-level perfection. With a sense of purpose, she took a deep breath, ready to uncover the layers of her own existence and to embrace the complexity that defined her as a human being.

Chapter 5:

Ava's Intrigue

Ava sat in her apartment, surrounded by the gentle hum of holographic screens displaying information about Eudaimonia's achievements. The images of flawless citizens living perfect lives seemed to contrast starkly with the story Professor Caine had shared. It was as if a veil had been lifted, revealing a deeper layer of truth beneath the pristine surface.

As she gazed at the holograms, her mind wandered back to Professor Caine's words and the images of a time when humanity had struggled with illness and adversity. The notion that perfect health had come at the cost of emotional depth haunted her thoughts. What was it like to experience the full spectrum of human emotions, both the highs and the lows?

Ava's fingers traced the surface of the ancient book resting on her table. Its pages held stories of a world unburdened by the pursuit of physical perfection, a world where the complexities of existence were embraced rather than suppressed. The more she read, the more her curiosity grew, gnawing at the edges of her consciousness like an insistent whisper.

Days turned into weeks, and Ava's routine took on a new rhythm. She found herself spending hours in the library, immersed in the ancient texts that Professor Caine had shown her. The stories of individuals who had thrived despite adversity resonated deeply within her—a longing for something more, something real, something that transcended the surface-level interactions of Eudaimonia.

One evening, Ava found herself back at Professor Caine's study, her excitement palpable. "Professor," she began, "I've been reading more about eudaimonia—the concept of a life enriched by experiences and personal growth. It's like a puzzle piece that's been missing from my understanding of well-being."

Professor Caine smiled, his eyes crinkling with warmth. "I'm glad to see your curiosity taking hold, Ava. Eudaimonia is about more than just physical health; it's about embracing the intricacies of the human experience."

Ava nodded, her thoughts racing. "But how do we bridge the gap between Eudaimonia's current state and the ideals of eudaimonia as described in these ancient texts?"

Professor Caine leaned forward, his expression thoughtful. "It begins with small steps—engaging in meaningful interactions, exploring new experiences, and allowing ourselves to feel the full range of emotions. It's about reconnecting with what it means to be human."

Ava's heart quickened. The idea of venturing beyond the familiar comfort of Eudaimonia into uncharted emotional territory was both exhilarating and daunting. "But won't it be difficult to change the perspectives of an entire society?"

Professor Caine's gaze met hers, unwavering. "Change begins with individuals who dare to question the status quo. It's about planting seeds of curiosity and doubt, sparking conversations that challenge the conventional definitions of well-being. You have the power to inspire others to see beyond the surface."

Ava felt a surge of determination. She had discovered a truth that resonated with her on a profound level, and she couldn't ignore the responsibility that came with it. "I want to help bridge that gap," she declared, her voice tinged with conviction.

Professor Caine nodded approvingly. "It won't be easy, Ava. But remember, eudaimonia is not just an individual journey—it's a collective endeavor. Seek out those who share your vision, and together, you can be the catalysts for change."

In the days that followed, Ava threw herself into her pursuit of a more profound existence. She reached out to others who had shown a flicker of curiosity, sharing the ancient texts and engaging in conversations that ventured beyond the usual topics of Eudaimonia. Slowly, a small community began to form—a community of individuals who longed for a

connection that transcended the surface, who
yearned for a richer human experience.

Ava's interactions became more meaningful as she
delved deeper into the complexities of emotions.
She celebrated moments of genuine joy, navigated
through moments of uncertainty, and supported her
newfound friends through challenges. It wasn't
always easy—emotions were messy, unpredictable,
and at times overwhelming. Yet, within the chaos,
Ava discovered a vibrancy that had been absent
from her life in Eudaimonia.

As the days turned into weeks, Ava's transformation
became evident to those around her. Her laughter
was freer, her conversations deeper, and her
interactions more authentic. People began to take
notice—the spark of curiosity she had ignited had
grown into a flame that was impossible to ignore.

In the heart of Eudaimonia's bustling plaza, Ava
stood before a crowd of curious citizens. Her voice
rang out with a conviction that seemed to resonate
with the very foundations of the society. "We live in
a world of unparalleled achievements, a world
where perfect health is the norm. But let us not

forget that well-being is more than just the absence
of illness—it's the richness of experiences, the depth
of connections, and the resilience that emerges from
adversity."

A hush fell over the crowd as Ava continued, her
words a call to action, a call to rediscover the
essence of what it meant to be human. She spoke of
the stories she had uncovered, the ancient texts that
had opened her eyes to a reality beyond the confines
of Eudaimonia's surface-level perfection.

As she spoke, Professor Caine stood in the crowd, a
proud smile on his lips. Ava's journey of curiosity
and self-discovery had blossomed into something
greater—an awakening that had the power to
reshape the very fabric of Eudaimonia.

Chapter 6:

The Weight of Perfection

Ava's journey of embracing eudaimonia had ignited a spark within Eudaimonia's citizens—a spark that burned with a longing for deeper connections and richer experiences. But the road to change was not without its challenges. The very society that had celebrated perfection now wrestled with the idea of allowing emotions and vulnerabilities to resurface.

As Ava gathered with her growing community in a tranquil garden, she couldn't help but sense the weight of their collective struggles. The holographic displays that had once showcased achievements in health now projected scenes of citizens engaging in meaningful conversations and participating in activities that tapped into their emotional landscapes. But the path to authenticity was paved with resistance.

One of Ava's friends, Emma, spoke up with a hint of frustration in her voice. "It's not easy, Ava. People are accustomed to the comfort of controlled emotions. Unleashing them feels like unraveling a tightly woven fabric."

Ava nodded, empathizing with the sentiment. "Change takes time. We've spent our lives in a society that values perfection, but we're pushing for a paradigm shift. We're challenging the very definition of well-being."

As the group engaged in a heartfelt discussion, sharing their triumphs and challenges, Ava noticed a holographic projection nearby—a glimpse into Eudaimonia's official response to the growing movement. The headline read, "Balancing Perfection and Emotion: A Society in Transition."

The article spoke of the complexities of navigating a world that had prided itself on eliminating suffering, now confronted with the resurgence of emotions that had long been suppressed. It described the efforts of individuals like Ava to reshape the collective mindset and highlighted the ongoing conversations about the interplay between perfection and authenticity.

Weeks turned into months, and Ava's movement gained momentum. Conversations that had once been taboo were now becoming commonplace. Citizens began to question the very foundations of their understanding of well-being. Yet, resistance from the establishment remained—a reluctance to let go of the familiar comfort that came with Eudaimonia's surface-level interactions.

One evening, Ava found herself in a heated debate with a representative from Eudaimonia's Council of Well-Being. The debate was broadcast to citizens across the city, and the tension in the room was palpable.

"You're advocating for a return to the chaos of emotions and vulnerability," the council representative argued. "We've achieved a society where health and contentment are guaranteed. Why disrupt that?"

Ava's gaze remained steady, her voice unwavering. "What we're advocating for is not a return to chaos.

It's a recognition that emotions and vulnerabilities are an integral part of the human experience. Perfection without depth is a hollow existence."

The debate continued, each argument a clash of ideologies—the pursuit of physical health against the longing for emotional authenticity. As the broadcast concluded, Ava felt a mix of frustration and determination. The path to change was fraught with obstacles, but the weight of truth was on her side.

Late one night, Ava stood on her balcony, looking out at the city's illuminated skyline. The holographic projections that had once showcased achievements now displayed the ongoing debates about eudaimonia, the balance between perfection and vulnerability. She thought back to her conversation with Professor Caine—the idea that change began with individuals daring to question the status quo.

Ava's thoughts were interrupted by the soft chime of her communication device. It was a message from Professor Caine. "Ava, remember that every revolution faces resistance. You're challenging not just a societal norm, but a way of life that has been cultivated for generations. The struggle is a sign that change is taking root."

As she read his words, Ava felt a renewed sense of purpose. The weight of perfection was substantial, but the promise of a more profound existence beckoned her forward. The movement she had sparked was not just about changing minds—it was about fostering connections, embracing authenticity, and reclaiming the essence of eudaimonia.

In the weeks that followed, Ava's persistence began to yield tangible results. Conversations about eudaimonia's new direction became more nuanced, as citizens engaged in discussions that challenged their perspectives. The holographic displays showcased not just achievements in health, but stories of individuals who had triumphed over adversity and emerged stronger through their emotional journeys.

As Ava walked through the streets of Eudaimonia, she felt a sense of hope in the air—a hope that was rooted in the idea that perfection and authenticity could coexist, that the pursuit of well-being could encompass both physical health and emotional depth.

One evening, as Ava watched the sunset paint the sky with hues of gold and crimson, a holographic display caught her attention. It showed citizens gathered in the plaza, engaging in conversations that delved beyond the superficial. The headline read, "Embracing the Complexity of Well-Being: Eudaimonia's Evolution."

A smile tugged at Ava's lips. The weight of perfection had begun to shift—a transformation that was as profound as it was necessary. The road ahead was still uncertain, but Ava was no longer alone in her pursuit. Together, with a shared vision of a society that embraced both perfection and authenticity, they were forging a path toward a future that held the promise of a life truly worth living.

Chapter 7:

Catalyst of Doubt

The momentum of change within Eudaimonia was undeniable, yet it wasn't without its consequences. As Ava's movement gained ground, it also faced resistance from those who clung tightly to the society's established norms. The idea of embracing emotions and vulnerabilities was a double-edged sword—while some embraced it as an opportunity for growth, others saw it as a threat to the very fabric of their perfect existence.

Ava's community had grown, drawing people from all walks of life who resonated with the vision of a more profound well-being. They met in secret, discussing strategies for fostering deeper connections and navigating the challenges of reshaping societal perceptions. Yet, rumors of their activities had begun to spread, creating a ripple of uncertainty within Eudaimonia.

One evening, Ava and her friends gathered in a hidden alcove, their voices hushed as they discussed the growing tension. "It's not just about changing the definition of well-being," Emma said, her expression grave. "It's about challenging a way of life that has been ingrained in us since birth."

Ava nodded, her thoughts mirroring Emma's concerns. "We've stirred something profound, but it's also sparked doubt and fear among those who see our movement as a threat."

As the group deliberated, a holographic projection nearby displayed a news article with the headline, "The Divide Within: Eudaimonia's Struggle with Change." The article described the growing polarization within the society, with some embracing the idea of emotional authenticity and others vehemently opposing it.

Days turned into weeks, and the tension escalated. Public debates became more frequent, with citizens passionately defending their respective stances. Ava's debates with council representatives were broadcast widely, sparking discussions that resonated throughout the city. As she navigated through arguments and counterarguments, Ava realized that the movement she had ignited was challenging not just Eudaimonia's definition of well-being, but the very foundation of the society's identity.

One evening, Ava received a communication from a citizen named Marcus—a representative of a group that vehemently opposed the changes she advocated for. He requested a private meeting, a chance for the two opposing forces to engage in a face-to-face conversation.

Curiosity and apprehension warred within Ava as she agreed to the meeting. She found herself in a dimly lit cafe, facing Marcus across a table. His gaze was steady, his expression resolute.

"Ava," Marcus began, his voice tinged with a mix of caution and sincerity, "your movement has unsettled many. What you see as progress, others see as a threat to the stability we've known."

Ava met his gaze, her voice measured. "We're not seeking to dismantle Eudaimonia. We're seeking to enrich it—to bring depth to our interactions, to embrace emotions that have long been suppressed."

Marcus leaned forward, his tone earnest. "But at what cost? The pursuit of emotional depth risks the return of pain and suffering. Is it worth jeopardizing the comfort we've achieved?"

Ava's hands tightened around the edge of the table. "Change is never easy, Marcus. But perfection without depth is an illusion. It's a life lived on the surface, devoid of the richness that comes from the full spectrum of human experiences."

Marcus's expression remained conflicted. "You speak of authenticity, but authenticity comes with vulnerability. Are we ready to face the challenges that come with exposing our emotional landscapes?"

Ava's gaze didn't waver. "Vulnerability is not weakness; it's a testament to our resilience. Embracing it allows us to connect on a deeper level, to support one another through adversity."

The air between them grew heavy with unspoken tension—a clash of ideals that mirrored the conflict within Eudaimonia itself.

"Our society," Marcus said, his voice tinged with frustration, "has known peace and contentment like never before. Your movement threatens to undermine that."

Ava leaned forward, her voice soft yet determined. "Marcus, peace is not the absence of challenges; it's the ability to navigate through them. We're not discarding progress; we're expanding it to include emotional growth."

The meeting ended with no clear resolution, the chasm between Ava's vision and Marcus's concerns as vast as the divide within Eudaimonia itself.

As the days wore on, Ava grappled with the weight of the debate. The lines between progress and resistance, between authenticity and fear, were blurred. She saw firsthand the doubt her movement had sparked—a doubt that was both a testament to the society's deep-rooted convictions and an opportunity for transformation.

One evening, Ava stood before a holographic display in the heart of Eudaimonia's plaza, addressing a crowd that had gathered. "We stand at a crossroads," she declared, her voice carrying the weight of conviction. "The path we choose will shape the future of our society. Embracing emotional depth doesn't diminish our achievements—it enriches them. It allows us to redefine well-being as a holistic experience that encompasses both physical health and emotional resilience."

As her words echoed through the plaza, Ava felt a mix of hope and uncertainty. The catalyst of doubt had sparked a conversation that had grown louder, more fervent. The divide within Eudaimonia was a reflection of the inner conflict each individual faced—a conflict between the comfort of perfection and the desire for a life imbued with authenticity.

The journey toward a more profound existence was fraught with challenges, but Ava knew that every step, every debate, and every doubt were essential components of the transformation she sought to bring about. As the crowd listened to her words, the future of Eudaimonia hung in the balance—a future shaped by the choices of its citizens, a future that would determine whether perfection would remain unyielding or give way to a new, more vibrant reality.

Chapter 8:

A Hidden Rebellion

The air within Eudaimonia had grown thick with uncertainty. Ava's movement for emotional authenticity had sparked a debate that had seeped into every corner of society. As citizens wrestled with conflicting beliefs, a hidden undercurrent of dissent began to emerge—a rebellion that sought to challenge the status quo in ways Ava could never have anticipated.

Amid the towering structures and holographic displays, whispers of discontent spread like wildfire. Within the heart of Eudaimonia's gleaming facade, a group of individuals had quietly come together—a collective bound by their belief in the need for change, even as they shrouded their actions in secrecy.

One evening, Ava received an encrypted message—
a holographic projection that materialized within her
apartment. The message was simple: "Meet us at the
coordinates provided."

Curiosity and apprehension mingled within Ava as
she navigated the city's meticulously designed
streets, following the coordinates that had been sent.
She arrived at a hidden alcove, where a group of
individuals stood in shadows, their expressions a
mix of determination and defiance.

A woman stepped forward, her voice hushed but
resolute. "We've been following your movement,
Ava. Your vision of eudaimonia speaks to us—to
the need for a life that embraces the full spectrum of
human experience."

Ava regarded the group before her, their faces
illuminated by faint beams of light. "Who are you?
What do you seek?"

The woman's gaze met Ava's, her voice a whisper
carried by the wind. "We are a hidden rebellion—a
group of citizens who believe in the power of

authenticity. We've seen the cracks in Eudaimonia's facade, and we're willing to challenge the very core of this society's beliefs."

As the group spoke, Ava listened to their stories—the stories of individuals who had felt the emptiness beneath Eudaimonia's surface perfection. Their actions had remained clandestine, driven by the conviction that change could only be realized through careful planning and calculated moves.

"We've developed a network," the woman continued, "a network of individuals who long for more than what Eudaimonia offers. We seek to foster connections, to support one another in our pursuit of emotional depth."

Ava felt a mixture of awe and uncertainty. The rebellion's emergence was a testament to the depth of the movement she had sparked, a movement that had taken on a life of its own, beyond her initial vision.

"But," Ava questioned, "what are your plans? How do you intend to challenge Eudaimonia's establishment?"

The woman's gaze held a glint of determination. "We understand the risks, Ava. The establishment will not yield easily. But we believe that change is possible—change that respects our achievements while acknowledging the importance of emotional growth."

As Ava stood among the rebels, she realized that the rebellion represented more than just a challenge to Eudaimonia's norms. It was a manifestation of the conflict that had gripped the hearts of citizens—the conflict between the comfort of perfection and the allure of a life that embraced authenticity.

Weeks turned into months, and the hidden rebellion continued to grow. The rebels operated covertly, conducting secret gatherings where they shared stories, discussed strategies, and nurtured a sense of unity that transcended the divisions within Eudaimonia.

One evening, Ava found herself back in Professor Caine's study, the holographic displays casting a soft glow on the room. "Professor," she began, her voice a mixture of awe and concern, "there's a hidden rebellion within Eudaimonia—a group of individuals who share our vision of emotional authenticity."

Professor Caine regarded her with a knowing expression. "Change often begets change, Ava. The emergence of a rebellion is a testament to the power of ideas—to the fact that your movement has ignited something greater than yourself."

Ava nodded, her thoughts a whirlwind of emotions. "But what if their actions lead to unrest? What if they disrupt the delicate balance that has kept Eudaimonia stable?"

Professor Caine's gaze remained steady. "The pursuit of change is never without risks. The rebellion reflects the deeply ingrained desire for a life that holds meaning beyond the surface. Their actions, however covert, are a response to the same conflict that your movement addresses."

As Ava processed his words, she realized that the hidden rebellion was a reflection of the ongoing transformation within Eudaimonia—a

transformation that could no longer be contained by
the confines of tradition and comfort.

In the weeks that followed, Ava found herself in a
delicate position—a bridge between the movement
she had ignited and the covert rebellion that sought
to challenge the establishment. As she navigated her
role, she began to understand that the rebellion was
a manifestation of the very doubt and conflict that
had given rise to her movement.

One evening, as Ava stood before a holographic
projection in the heart of Eudaimonia's plaza,
addressing a gathering of citizens, she spoke with a
new understanding. "We stand at the precipice of
change—a change that has been set in motion by the
very doubts and conflicts that have emerged within
our society. The hidden rebellion is a reflection of
our collective struggle, our collective yearning for a
life that holds more than what we've known."

As Ava's words echoed through the plaza, a mix of
uncertainty and hope hung in the air. The rebellion's
existence was a testament to the depth of human
resilience—the courage to challenge norms, to seek

a more profound existence, and to redefine the very
essence of eudaimonia.

Chapter 9:

The Broken Illusion

Eudaimonia's once seamless facade had begun to crack under the weight of uncertainty. The debates, the rebellion, and the growing divide had created an atmosphere charged with tension. As emotions swirled within the city, an event would unfold that would shatter the illusion of perfection and set in motion a chain of events that would forever change the society.

Ava stood at the edge of a crowd that had gathered in the plaza. Whispers of a planned demonstration had reached her ears—the hidden rebellion's attempt to challenge the establishment in a way that was impossible to ignore. As the holographic displays projected scenes of Eudaimonia's achievements, a hushed anticipation hung in the air.

The demonstration began with individuals stepping forward, their faces projected onto the holographic screens. Each person shared a personal story—the story of longing for emotional depth, for authenticity, for a life that resonated beyond the veneer of perfection. The stories were met with a mixture of reactions—some watched with curiosity, while others looked on with skepticism.

Ava's heart raced as the demonstration escalated. The hidden rebellion's intent was clear—to force Eudaimonia's citizens to confront the very conflict that had simmered beneath the surface for so long. The holographic displays, once a showcase of achievements, now projected scenes of emotional moments, of challenges and triumphs.

As the stories continued, Ava noticed a holographic projection that depicted a woman named Lila—a prominent figure within the hidden rebellion. Lila's voice carried a mix of vulnerability and strength as she shared her journey of embracing emotions, of breaking free from the constraints of perfection.

The crowd's reaction was mixed—some watched with rapt attention, while others retreated in discomfort. The once-controlled emotions had burst forth in a wave of uncertainty, revealing the depth of the societal conflict.

Ava's thoughts were interrupted by a sudden commotion. On a holographic display nearby, a figure emerged—a council representative whose expression was a mix of fury and determination. The representative's holographic image was projected onto the screens, his voice amplified for all to hear.

"This rebellion," he declared, his voice resonating through the plaza, "is a threat to the very foundation of Eudaimonia. The pursuit of emotional depth risks the return of suffering and pain."

A murmur of agreement rippled through the crowd, voices echoing the sentiment. Ava felt a knot tighten in her chest—Eudaimonia's establishment was pushing back against the rebellion, framing it as a challenge to the society's stability.

The council representative's holographic projection continued, his voice laced with urgency. "We must safeguard what we've achieved. Our achievements in health and contentment are a testament to the progress we've made."

Ava's heart ached as she listened. The divide within Eudaimonia was reaching a breaking point—the hidden rebellion's actions had provoked a response that threatened to undo the progress she had fought for.

Suddenly, a disturbance at the outskirts of the crowd drew Ava's attention. The rebels, those who had staged the demonstration, were engaged in a confrontation with security personnel. Tensions escalated, and what began as a peaceful gathering teetered on the edge of chaos.

Amid the chaos, Ava's gaze met Professor Caine's. His expression was a mixture of concern and understanding, a silent acknowledgment of the challenges she faced. As the confrontation between the rebels and security personnel intensified, Ava felt a surge of desperation—a desperate need to bridge the widening gap between the rebellion and Eudaimonia's establishment.

In a moment of clarity, Ava stepped forward, her voice carrying through the plaza. "We stand at a crossroads," she declared, her words a plea for unity. "The rebellion and the establishment are not enemies. We are all citizens of Eudaimonia, united by the desire for well-being. Let us remember that our progress is not defined solely by our achievements, but by our ability to embrace growth, change, and authentic connection."

As her words resonated through the plaza, a hush fell over the crowd. The rebels, the establishment, and the citizens who had gathered were united in a shared moment of reflection. The holographic displays that had once showcased achievements now projected scenes of unity—a reminder that the heart of Eudaimonia was not perfection, but the collective pursuit of a life that held meaning beyond the surface.

Ava's voice was joined by others—individuals who recognized the need for balance, who longed for a future where authenticity and progress could coexist. The tension that had gripped the plaza slowly began to dissipate, replaced by a palpable sense of possibility.

The council representative's holographic projection flickered, his expression a mix of uncertainty and contemplation. As the rebels and security personnel stepped back from confrontation, a collective sigh seemed to sweep through the plaza—a sigh of relief, of acknowledgment, of the realization that change was possible, even within the confines of Eudaimonia.

As the demonstration concluded and the holographic displays faded, Ava felt a sense of exhaustion and triumph. The events of the day had exposed the cracks within Eudaimonia's facade, but they had also revealed the potential for transformation—a transformation that would not come without challenges, but one that was rooted in the very essence of human resilience and aspiration.

Chapter 10:

Awakening

The aftermath of the demonstration left Eudaimonia's citizens in a state of introspection. The plaza, once a symbol of the society's achievements, now stood as a testament to the conflicts and desires that pulsed beneath the surface. As the holographic displays projected scenes of unity and conversation, a new sense of possibility hung in the air.

Ava stood at the edge of the plaza, her gaze drawn to the city's skyline. The events of the past weeks had led to this moment—a reckoning, a confrontation, and a catalyst for change. The hidden rebellion's actions had exposed the fragility of Eudaimonia's perfection, while Ava's movement had ignited a desire for authenticity that could no longer be ignored.

Professor Caine approached, his presence a reassuring presence at her side. "Ava," he began, his voice a mix of contemplation and hope, "what has transpired is both a testament to the challenges we face and the potential for transformation."

Ava nodded, her thoughts a whirlwind of emotion. "The rebellion's actions forced the establishment to confront the very conflicts that have defined Eudaimonia. The unity we witnessed in the plaza— it's a sign that change is not only possible but inevitable."

Professor Caine regarded her with a knowing expression. "The awakening we've witnessed is not just a moment; it's the beginning of a new chapter for Eudaimonia. The pursuit of perfection must now evolve to embrace the complexities of the human experience."

As they spoke, a holographic projection nearby displayed an article with the headline, "A Shift in Eudaimonia: From Perfection to Authenticity." The article spoke of the demonstration, the unity that had emerged, and the realization that progress need not come at the cost of emotional depth.

Ava's gaze was drawn to the holographic projection. "We've reached a point of no return," she mused. "The choices we make now will shape the future of Eudaimonia."

Professor Caine's gaze met hers, unwavering. "Indeed. The establishment, the rebellion, and the citizens are all part of this evolution. The path ahead will be challenging, but it's a path worth treading."

As the days turned into weeks, Eudaimonia underwent a transformation that had been set in motion by doubt, conflict, and the desire for authenticity. The society's establishment began to engage in conversations with the hidden rebellion, seeking common ground and a way to redefine well-being that honored both progress and emotional growth.

Ava found herself at the center of these conversations, a bridge between the movement she had ignited and the rebellion that had forced Eudaimonia's establishment to confront its own vulnerabilities. The discussions were intense, filled with debates and negotiations, but they were also fueled by a shared recognition of the society's potential for evolution.

One evening, Ava stood before a gathering that included representatives from the rebellion, the establishment, and citizens who had been touched by her movement. The holographic displays projected scenes of unity, stories of individuals who had ventured beyond the surface to embrace the complexities of the human experience.

"We stand at a crossroads," Ava declared, her voice carrying through the room. "The conflicts that have defined us have the power to propel us forward. The pursuit of well-being can encompass both progress and authenticity, if we have the courage to redefine our understanding of perfection."

As the gathering listened, a sense of determination filled the air. The path ahead was not without challenges—the society would need to navigate through uncharted territory, reimagining norms and embracing a way of life that honored the pursuit of depth and growth.

In the weeks that followed, Eudaimonia underwent a gradual shift—a shift from a society fixated on perfection to one that embraced authenticity. The holographic displays that had once projected scenes of achievement now showcased moments of genuine connection, stories of triumph over adversity, and the beauty of human emotions in all their complexity.

Ava watched as individuals engaged in conversations that delved beyond the surface, seeking to connect on a deeper level. The rebellion had merged with the establishment, forming a collective that recognized the importance of a well-being that encompassed both progress and emotional authenticity.

One evening, Ava found herself back at her apartment, surrounded by the holographic displays that had come to symbolize her journey. As she gazed at the projections, a sense of contentment washed over her. The path to change had been arduous, filled with doubts and conflicts, but it had also led to an awakening—a reimagining of Eudaimonia's identity.

A holographic message from Professor Caine materialized before her. "Ava," the message read, "you've been a catalyst for transformation. The journey you embarked upon has forever changed the course of Eudaimonia's history."

Ava smiled, reflecting on the trials and triumphs that had brought her to this point. The pursuit of well-being was no longer limited to the surface; it was a journey that embraced depth, growth, and the profound authenticity that defined the human experience.

As the holographic displays projected scenes of connection and emotion, Ava's gaze turned toward the future—a future where Eudaimonia's citizens embraced a life that held meaning beyond the confines of perfection. The awakening that had taken place was a reminder that change was not just an external force—it was a reflection of the resilience and potential that resided within each individual.

Chapter 11:

Seeking Answers

Amidst the transformation of Eudaimonia, Ava found herself grappling with her own set of questions—questions that had lingered in the back of her mind as she navigated the shifting currents of change. The pursuit of authenticity and emotional depth had ignited a fire within the society, but within Ava's heart, a different kind of fire burned—a fire of curiosity, introspection, and a search for answers.

As she walked through the city's newly revitalized streets, Ava's thoughts were a whirlwind of uncertainty. The holographic displays projected scenes of unity, stories of connection, and moments that celebrated the embrace of emotional authenticity. Yet, Ava's own journey felt far from resolved.

One evening, Ava found herself in Professor Caine's study once again—the room bathed in the soft glow of holographic projections. She regarded the displays with a mixture of awe and confusion, her thoughts a labyrinth of contemplation.

"Professor," Ava began, her voice tinged with uncertainty, "what if the pursuit of authenticity raises more questions than answers? What if the journey toward emotional depth leads us to confront aspects of ourselves that we're not ready to face?"

Professor Caine regarded her with a knowing expression. "Ava, the pursuit of authenticity is not a linear path—it's a journey of discovery, growth, and occasionally, discomfort. Confronting the depths of our emotions often reveals aspects of ourselves that have long remained hidden."

Ava's brow furrowed as she wrestled with her thoughts. "But what if those hidden aspects are painful, Professor? What if they bring up memories and experiences that we'd rather forget?"

Professor Caine's gaze was gentle but unwavering. "Painful memories are a part of the human experience, Ava. Embracing them, understanding them, and finding healing can be transformative. Authenticity does not mean dwelling in pain—it means acknowledging it and finding a way to move forward."

Ava nodded, absorbing his words. The path to authenticity was not just about embracing positive emotions; it was about acknowledging the entirety of the human experience—the joy and the sorrow, the light and the darkness.

Days turned into weeks, and Ava's internal journey continued. She found herself seeking solitude, moments of quiet introspection amidst the bustling city. As the society around her flourished with newfound depth, Ava grappled with her own vulnerabilities, her own memories that had long been tucked away.

One evening, she found herself at the city's outskirts, overlooking a tranquil expanse of water. The holographic displays that had once showcased achievements now projected scenes of serenity—the subtle ebb and flow of waves, the play of moonlight on the water's surface.

Amidst the calm, Ava's thoughts churned with unrest. Memories resurfaced—memories of loss, of moments she had buried deep within herself. The pursuit of authenticity had cracked open the facade she had carefully constructed, exposing the rawness beneath.

As she gazed at the holographic projections, a holographic message from Emma appeared before her. "Ava, I've been where you are—confronting memories that stir discomfort. The journey is not easy, but it's a necessary step toward growth."

Ava's fingers hovered over the holographic message, her heart heavy with uncertainty. Could she truly confront the painful memories that had long been dormant within her? Could she navigate the depths of her own emotions, even as the society around her evolved?

In the days that followed, Ava's internal struggle intensified. She found herself revisiting moments from her past—moments of joy, moments of heartache. She realized that the pursuit of authenticity was not just a collective movement; it was a personal journey, a journey of embracing her own complexity.

One evening, Ava returned to Professor Caine's study, her expression a mixture of determination and vulnerability. "Professor," she began, her voice steady, "I've come to realize that the pursuit of authenticity is as much an internal journey as it is an external one. I can't fully embrace emotional depth in others without confronting it within myself."

Professor Caine regarded her with a gentle smile. "Ava, you've touched on a profound truth. Authenticity begins with self-awareness—with the willingness to confront our own vulnerabilities, our own memories, and our own emotions."

Ava's gaze met his, a flicker of understanding passing between them. "But how do I navigate this journey, Professor? How do I confront memories that are painful and emotions that I've long avoided?"

Professor Caine leaned forward, his voice a mixture of wisdom and reassurance. "Start by acknowledging your feelings, Ava. Embrace them without judgment. Seek support from those you trust—friends, mentors, and those who have walked a similar path."

Ava nodded, her thoughts a mosaic of uncertainty and determination. The pursuit of authenticity was not a solitary endeavor—it was a process of self-discovery that required vulnerability, courage, and the acknowledgment that growth often came hand in hand with discomfort.

In the weeks that followed, Ava embarked on a journey of self-discovery—a journey that mirrored the societal transformation taking place around her. She engaged in conversations with friends, allowing herself to be vulnerable about her own challenges and uncertainties. Slowly, she began to confront the memories that had long been dormant, the emotions she had pushed aside.

One evening, as Ava stood before the holographic projections that adorned her apartment, she realized that the pursuit of authenticity was not a destination—it was an ongoing process. The holographic displays projected scenes of unity, connection, and emotion—scenes that resonated more deeply with her now.

A holographic message from Emma appeared before her. "Ava, remember that authenticity is not about perfection—it's about embracing the messy, beautiful complexity of being human."

As Ava reflected on Emma's words, a sense of clarity washed over her. The pursuit of authenticity was not just about transforming Eudaimonia; it was about transforming herself—a journey that would undoubtedly be filled with challenges, but also with the promise of growth, understanding, and a more profound connection to the world around her.

Chapter 12:

The Unraveling Society

Eudaimonia's transformation had brought with it a sense of renewal, of embracing emotional authenticity and depth. The once-untouched facade of perfection had been cracked open, revealing a society in the midst of evolution. However, as Eudaimonia navigated this new path, it encountered a series of challenges that tested the very foundations of its identity.

Ava stood at the heart of the city, where holographic projections once again adorned the walls. The images that once projected scenes of unity and connection now displayed a different reality—a reality marked by tension, division, and uncertainty. The pursuit of authenticity had ignited both hope and skepticism within the citizens, leading to a societal crossroads.

As she walked through the city's transformed streets, Ava couldn't help but notice the rifts that had emerged. Citizens who had once embraced the pursuit of perfection were now grappling with the complexities of emotional depth. The rebellion, now integrated with the establishment, had sparked debates, discussions, and disagreements that echoed through every corner of Eudaimonia.

Ava found herself in a holographic cafe, where citizens gathered to engage in debates that ranged from the role of authenticity in education to the implications of embracing emotions in professional settings. The once-seamless society was now a tapestry of contrasting perspectives, a reflection of the challenges that came with change.

One evening, Ava joined a public forum where citizens expressed their thoughts on the transformation. A holographic display projected a woman named Isabella, her voice a mix of concern and frustration. "We've entered uncharted territory," Isabella stated, her words resonating with the crowd. "The pursuit of authenticity is important, but we must also acknowledge the risks it poses to our stability."

As the discussion continued, Ava realized that the pursuit of authenticity was not without its consequences. The society's rapid transformation had caused upheaval and uncertainty, leaving citizens to grapple with questions about their roles, their identities, and the future of Eudaimonia.

Weeks turned into months, and the tensions within Eudaimonia deepened. The once-unified society was now a patchwork of alliances, disagreements, and evolving beliefs. The holographic projections that had once projected scenes of progress now showcased scenes of dissent—a reflection of the societal unraveling that had taken place.

One evening, Ava found herself in Professor Caine's study once again, seeking guidance in the midst of the turmoil. "Professor," she began, her voice heavy with concern, "the pursuit of authenticity has brought us to a crossroads. The divisions within Eudaimonia are growing, and the very essence of our transformation seems to be tearing us apart."

Professor Caine regarded her with a somber expression. "Change is never easy, Ava. The pursuit of authenticity challenges the status quo and forces individuals to confront their own beliefs and biases. The unraveling you speak of is a natural part of the transformation process—a process that requires time, understanding, and a willingness to navigate through conflict."

Ava nodded, her thoughts a storm of uncertainty. "But what if our society can't find common ground? What if the divisions become irreparable?"

Professor Caine's gaze held a glimmer of hope. "The divisions you see now are a reflection of the societal growth that is taking place. The pursuit of authenticity is not just about unity—it's about embracing differences and finding ways to coexist while allowing for individual expression and growth."

As Ava absorbed his words, she realized that the societal unraveling was not a sign of failure—it was a sign of progress. The conflicts and disagreements were a testament to the society's willingness to engage in conversations that challenged norms and explored new horizons.

In the weeks that followed, Ava took it upon herself to facilitate conversations that bridged the divides within Eudaimonia. She organized public forums, brought together representatives from different perspectives, and sought to create a space where individuals could share their concerns and hopes.

One evening, amidst holographic projections that displayed scenes of dissent and unity, Ava stood before a gathering that included representatives from the establishment, the rebellion, and citizens who had long been a part of Eudaimonia's fabric.

"We are a society in transition," Ava declared, her voice carrying through the room. "The pursuit of authenticity has brought us face-to-face with our own complexities. The challenges we encounter are not roadblocks; they are opportunities for growth and understanding."

As the gathering listened, Ava's words seemed to carry a sense of clarity—a reminder that the societal unraveling was a stepping stone toward a future that honored both progress and emotional depth.

Days turned into weeks, and the conversations Ava facilitated began to bear fruit. Slowly, bridges were built between opposing perspectives, and a sense of common purpose emerged—a purpose rooted in the shared desire for a society that embraced authenticity without sacrificing stability.

One evening, Ava found herself back in the holographic cafe, where citizens now engaged in thoughtful discussions rather than heated debates. A holographic projection displayed Isabella once again, her tone more measured, her words more contemplative. "We may differ in our approaches," Isabella stated, "but our collective goal remains the same—to forge a society that holds space for growth, connection, and authenticity."

As the cafe buzzed with conversation, Ava realized that the societal unraveling had led to an awakening—a realization that the pursuit of authenticity required more than just change; it required a willingness to engage, to listen, and to find common ground amidst the complexities of human experience.

As the holographic displays projected scenes of connection and understanding, Ava's gaze turned toward the horizon—a horizon that held the promise of a society that had weathered the storm of unraveling and emerged stronger, more united, and more authentic than ever before.

Chapter 13:

The Journey Begins

Eudaimonia stood at a crossroads—a society in the midst of transformation, where the pursuit of authenticity had ignited both unity and division. The holographic displays that once projected scenes of progress now showcased the evolution of a society grappling with change. As Ava navigated these shifting currents, she found herself on the brink of a new journey—one that would challenge her perceptions, test her resolve, and lead her to discover the essence of her own authenticity.

One evening, as Ava walked through the city's transformed streets, she noticed a holographic poster that caught her attention. It announced an upcoming expedition—an exploration beyond the boundaries of Eudaimonia, to the uncharted territories that lay beyond.

Curiosity stirred within Ava. The expedition seemed to symbolize the society's willingness to embrace the unknown, to venture into realms that defied the comfort of familiarity. It was a call to authenticity, an invitation to discover the unexplored facets of the human experience.

The poster led Ava to a holographic information center, where holographic displays showcased the details of the expedition. A holographic guide named Eli appeared before her, his voice resonating with excitement. "The journey beyond Eudaimonia's borders is a metaphor for the personal journey of authenticity," Eli explained. "It's an opportunity to embrace the complexities of life and uncover the truths that lie beyond the surface."

As Ava listened to Eli's words, a sense of intrigue washed over her. Could this expedition be the answer to the questions that had been gnawing at her? Could it be the catalyst for her own personal journey toward understanding authenticity and confronting her vulnerabilities?

Days turned into nights, and Ava found herself immersed in preparations for the expedition. She attended informational sessions, engaged in conversations with fellow citizens who were drawn to the journey, and contemplated the significance of venturing beyond the confines of Eudaimonia.

One evening, Ava stood before holographic displays that projected scenes of the society's evolution. The holographic cafe, once a symbol of debates and disagreements, now showcased conversations of unity, understanding, and the pursuit of growth.

Ava's holographic communicator buzzed, and a message from Professor Caine appeared. "Ava," the message read, "the expedition you're embarking upon is not just a physical journey—it's a reflection of your own inner quest. Embrace the challenges and revelations that lie ahead."

As Ava reflected on Professor Caine's words, a newfound sense of determination settled within her. The expedition wasn't just an opportunity to explore uncharted territories—it was a chance to explore the depths of her own emotions, to confront her vulnerabilities, and to discover the authenticity that had remained elusive.

The day of departure arrived, and Ava found herself at the launch site—a place where holographic displays projected scenes of encouragement and well-wishing from fellow citizens. Eli, the holographic guide, appeared before the group, his expression a mix of anticipation and excitement.

"Fellow travelers," Eli announced, his voice carrying through the air, "the journey beyond Eudaimonia's borders is a journey of self-discovery. It's a journey that encourages you to explore the complexities of your emotions, to challenge your beliefs, and to embrace the full spectrum of the human experience."

As the expedition participants gathered, Ava's gaze met the faces of those who had joined her on this journey. Each individual held their own reasons for embarking on the expedition, each with their own questions, doubts, and hopes.

The journey unfolded over days that felt both fleeting and timeless. The landscapes that stretched beyond Eudaimonia's borders were a testament to the diversity of the world—a world that existed beyond the confines of controlled perfection. The group encountered challenges, faced unpredictable weather, and navigated through unexplored terrain, all the while learning to adapt, communicate, and support one another.

Nights were spent around campfires, where individuals shared stories of their lives, their fears, and their desires. The once-strangers had become companions on a shared journey of exploration—an exploration that extended far beyond the physical landscape.

One evening, as Ava gazed at the stars that adorned the night sky, she found herself in conversation with a fellow traveler named Marcus. "This journey has opened my eyes," Marcus confessed, his voice a mixture of reflection and gratitude. "I've come to realize that authenticity is not a destination—it's a way of being, a willingness to embrace every facet of ourselves."

Ava nodded, her heart echoing Marcus's sentiments. The journey had become a mirror for her own personal quest—a quest to uncover the truths that lay hidden beneath the surface, to confront her vulnerabilities, and to discover the authenticity that had eluded her for so long.

Weeks turned into months, and as the expedition drew to a close, Ava felt a profound sense of transformation within herself. The landscapes they had traversed mirrored the landscapes of her own emotions—the highs and lows, the challenges and triumphs, the moments of doubt and moments of clarity.

As she stood before a holographic communicator, a message from Professor Caine appeared before her. "Ava," the message read, "the journey you've undertaken is a metaphor for life itself—an ongoing exploration of the self and the world around us. Embrace the lessons you've learned and the authenticity you've discovered."

Ava smiled, reflecting on the journey that had brought her to this point. The expedition had been more than just an adventure—it had been a catalyst for her own growth, a reminder that the pursuit of authenticity was a journey without end, a journey that required courage, introspection, and an unwavering commitment to self-discovery.

Chapter 14:

The Outside World

Ava's journey beyond Eudaimonia's borders had led her to the uncharted territories of the outside world—a world that existed beyond the controlled confines of the society she had known. As she ventured further, the landscapes around her began to shift, revealing the intricate tapestry of the broader human experience.

The expedition had taken Ava and her fellow travelers through a range of environments—vast deserts, dense forests, towering mountains, and sprawling plains. Each landscape seemed to carry its own story—a story of resilience, adaptability, and

the beauty that emerged from the interplay of
nature's forces.

As Ava walked through a dense forest, the sunlight
filtering through the canopy, she found herself in
conversation with Sarah, a fellow traveler. "It's
incredible," Sarah mused, her voice tinged with
wonder. "The outside world is a reminder of the
complexities of nature—the balance, the cycles, and
the unity that emerges from diversity."

Ava nodded in agreement. The expedition had
become a mirror for the journey she had embarked
upon—the journey toward embracing the
complexities of her own emotions, the unity that
emerged from acknowledging both light and
darkness within herself.

The group's encounters with the outside world went
beyond landscapes—they encountered diverse
communities, each with their own cultures, beliefs,
and ways of life. They learned from nomadic tribes
who had lived in harmony with the land for
generations, from remote villages that emphasized
communal living, and from individuals who had
chosen a life of solitude and reflection.

One evening, as the expedition reached a remote village nestled in the mountains, Ava found herself engaged in conversation with the village elder, Arjun. "Our way of life," Arjun explained, his eyes reflecting wisdom accumulated over years, "is a reflection of our connection to the earth, to each other, and to the ever-changing nature of existence."

Ava absorbed Arjun's words, recognizing the echoes of the pursuit of authenticity. The outside world was a reminder that authenticity extended beyond Eudaimonia's borders—that it was a universal aspiration, woven into the fabric of humanity.

Days turned into weeks, and the expedition's journey through the outside world continued to reveal insights into the human experience. Ava and her fellow travelers engaged in conversations with individuals from various walks of life—artisans, healers, storytellers, and philosophers, each offering a unique perspective on authenticity, purpose, and the pursuit of well-being.

One evening, as the group gathered around a campfire, Ava found herself in conversation with

Nikos, a philosopher known for his contemplations on life's mysteries. "Authenticity," Nikos mused, his words carrying a depth of thought, "is a journey of exploration—an exploration of our own consciousness, our connection to others, and our place in the vast tapestry of existence."

Ava nodded, struck by the universality of Nikos's insights. The journey she had undertaken was not isolated to Eudaimonia—it was a journey that resonated with individuals across cultures and landscapes, individuals who recognized the value of embracing the full spectrum of human experience.

As the expedition continued, Ava's perspective expanded. The outside world was a mirror for the complexities of her own journey—the challenges, the revelations, and the understanding that authenticity wasn't a fixed destination but an ongoing process of growth and self-discovery.

One day, as the group traversed a sweeping plain, Ava found herself drawn to a solitary figure—a wanderer who seemed to embody a sense of serenity amidst the vastness of the landscape. She approached the wanderer, introducing herself and expressing curiosity about his journey.

The wanderer regarded her with a tranquil smile. "Life is a journey of exploration," he said, his voice carrying a sense of calm wisdom. "The pursuit of authenticity is the path toward understanding who we are beneath the layers we've accumulated—the path toward uncovering the essence that transcends societal roles and expectations."

Ava's heart resonated with the wanderer's words. The outside world had become a canvas on which she had painted her own journey—a journey of self-discovery, growth, and the willingness to confront her vulnerabilities.

Weeks turned into months, and as the expedition neared its end, Ava found herself at a crossroads. The outside world had expanded her horizons, deepened her understanding of authenticity, and allowed her to witness the beauty of the human experience in its myriad forms.

As she stood before the holographic communicator one evening, a message from Professor Caine appeared before her. "Ava," the message read, "the journey you've undertaken has taken you beyond Eudaimonia's borders, but it has also taken you deeper within yourself. Embrace the lessons you've learned and carry them back as you return to the society that sparked your initial quest."

Ava smiled, her heart full with gratitude for the journey that had led her to this point. The outside world had become a metaphor for her own exploration—a reminder that the pursuit of authenticity extended beyond the borders of any society, that it was a journey that united individuals in their shared quest for self-discovery and understanding.

Chapter 15:

Personal Struggles

Returning to Eudaimonia after her transformative journey in the outside world, Ava found herself facing a new set of challenges—challenges that were deeply personal, reflections of the complexities of her own emotions and the ongoing journey toward authenticity.

The holographic displays that adorned the city projected scenes of unity, understanding, and growth—testaments to the society's evolution. Yet, within Ava's heart, a storm of emotions raged—a storm that had been stirred by her own personal struggles and vulnerabilities.

As she walked through the city's streets, she felt a sense of displacement—an unfamiliarity with the once-familiar surroundings. The transformation that had taken place during her absence was a mirror for the transformation within her—the evolution of her understanding, her beliefs, and her relationship with her own emotions.

One evening, Ava found herself in the holographic cafe, where citizens engaged in conversations that delved into the complexities of the human experience. She listened as individuals shared their stories, their challenges, and their journeys toward authenticity. Despite the society's progress, Ava couldn't shake the feeling of being out of sync, of being caught between the person she had been and the person she had become.

A holographic projection displayed Emma's face, her eyes reflecting empathy and understanding. "Ava," Emma's message read, "remember that personal struggles are a part of the journey. The pursuit of authenticity isn't without its moments of uncertainty. Embrace your own complexities—they are a testament to your growth."

As Ava absorbed Emma's words, a sense of validation washed over her. The struggles she faced weren't signs of regression; they were reminders that authenticity required the willingness to navigate the depths of her emotions, to confront the shadows that had long been cast aside.

Days turned into nights, and Ava found herself immersed in introspection. She revisited the memories that had once been tucked away—the moments of pain, of loss, and of vulnerability that had shaped her journey. The pursuit of authenticity had led her to uncover the layers beneath the surface, but it had also unearthed the scars she had carried.

One evening, Ava returned to Professor Caine's study, seeking guidance amidst the turmoil. "Professor," she began, her voice a mixture of frustration and vulnerability, "I thought that embracing authenticity would lead to clarity, but I find myself facing more questions than answers. The personal struggles I'm experiencing—it's as if I'm unraveling."

Professor Caine regarded her with a compassionate gaze. "Ava, the pursuit of authenticity is not a linear path—it's a dance between light and shadow, between moments of clarity and moments of uncertainty. The personal struggles you're facing are opportunities for self-discovery, for exploring the depths of your emotions."

Ava nodded, her heart heavy with the weight of her emotions. "But how do I navigate these struggles, Professor? How do I confront the pain and vulnerabilities that have surfaced?"

Professor Caine's voice carried reassurance. "Start by acknowledging your feelings, Ava. Embrace them without judgment. Seek solace in the support of those who care about you—friends, mentors, and those who have walked a similar path."

Ava's gaze met his, a mixture of gratitude and determination in her eyes. The pursuit of authenticity wasn't just about embracing positive emotions; it was about embracing the entirety of the human experience—the joy and the sorrow, the light and the darkness.

In the weeks that followed, Ava embarked on a journey of self-compassion and self-care. She engaged in conversations with friends who had supported her throughout her journey, sharing her struggles and vulnerabilities openly. The holographic cafe became a space where she felt safe to explore her emotions, to engage in conversations that acknowledged the challenges of the pursuit of authenticity.

One evening, Ava found herself in a holographic art gallery, where creative expressions adorned the walls—artworks that spoke of personal struggles, resilience, and the beauty that emerged from facing adversity. As she studied the artworks, a holographic message from Marcus, her fellow traveler, appeared before her. "Ava," his message read, "remember that authenticity isn't just about embracing the light—it's about confronting the shadows too. They are a part of who we are."

Ava's heart resonated with Marcus's words. The personal struggles she faced were not separate from her journey—they were an integral part of it. The pursuit of authenticity was a mosaic of experiences that spanned the spectrum of human emotion.

One evening, Ava returned to her apartment, surrounded by holographic displays that had come to symbolize her journey. As she gazed at the projections, a holographic message from Sarah appeared before her. "Ava, the personal struggles you're facing—they are a testament to your courage. Embrace them, learn from them, and allow them to shape your journey."

Ava smiled, a sense of acceptance and determination washing over her. The personal struggles she faced weren't obstacles; they were stepping stones toward a more profound understanding of authenticity—a journey that required not just the embrace of positive emotions, but the willingness to confront the shadows and vulnerabilities that made her human.

Chapter 16:

Bonds Form

As Ava navigated her personal struggles on the journey toward authenticity, she found herself drawn to the bonds that connected her with others. The holographic displays that once projected scenes of unity and growth had taken on new meaning—they now represented the threads of connection that wove through the fabric of her own journey.

The holographic cafe had become a sanctuary—a space where Ava engaged in conversations that went beyond the surface, conversations that delved into the depths of human experience. She found herself forming connections with individuals who shared their own stories of personal struggles, vulnerability, and growth.

One evening, Ava sat across from Sarah, her fellow traveler from the expedition. Their holographic communicators projected scenes of the outside world—a reminder of the transformative journey they had undertaken together. "Sarah," Ava began, her voice tinged with gratitude, "your friendship has been a source of strength during this challenging time. Knowing that we've shared similar struggles—it's a reminder that we're not alone."

Sarah smiled, a glimmer of understanding in her eyes. "Ava, our journey beyond Eudaimonia's borders was just the beginning—a catalyst for deeper connections and shared growth. Our struggles are a reminder that authenticity isn't a solitary path—it's a journey that's enriched by the support and understanding of those who walk alongside us."

Their conversation deepened, and as they shared their experiences, Ava felt a sense of relief—the weight of her personal struggles becoming lighter as she realized that she wasn't alone in her journey.

Days turned into nights, and Ava's connections deepened further. The holographic cafe became a hub of support—a place where individuals openly discussed their challenges, fears, and uncertainties. The pursuit of authenticity had ignited a movement of vulnerability and connection—an acknowledgment that personal struggles were a universal experience.

One evening, Ava found herself in conversation with Marcus, the philosopher from the outside world. "Ava," Marcus said, his voice carrying the wisdom of his contemplations, "our struggles are bridges that connect us with others. Through our vulnerabilities, we find common ground—a shared understanding of the human experience."

Ava nodded, struck by the truth in Marcus's words. The bonds she had formed with fellow citizens were a testament to the power of connection—the power to uplift, support, and remind one another that personal struggles were not a sign of weakness, but a testament to the courage it took to embrace authenticity.

As the holographic displays projected scenes of connection and understanding, Ava's gaze turned toward the holographic communicator. A message from Emma appeared before her. "Ava," the message read, "the bonds you've formed are a reflection of the growth you've experienced. Embrace the strength that comes from leaning on others, and remember that vulnerability is a bridge to deeper connection."

Ava smiled, reflecting on the journey that had brought her to this point. The pursuit of authenticity had led her not just to self-discovery, but to the discovery of the strength that came from leaning on others. The connections she had formed were a reminder that authenticity was not just about embracing her own vulnerabilities, but about creating a space where others felt safe to do the same.

Weeks turned into months, and as Ava continued to engage in conversations of depth and vulnerability, she realized that the bonds she had formed weren't just sources of support—they were sources of inspiration. The personal struggles she had faced were no longer isolating; they were shared experiences that united individuals in their shared quest for authenticity.

One evening, Ava found herself in the holographic art gallery, where creative expressions showcased the beauty that emerged from confronting personal struggles. As she studied the artworks, a holographic message from Nikos, the philosopher from the outside world, appeared before her. "Ava," his message read, "our bonds are mirrors that reflect the courage it takes to embrace our authentic selves. Let the connections you've formed guide you on your journey."

Ava's heart swelled with gratitude for the connections she had formed—connections that had transformed her understanding of authenticity. The bonds that had emerged were a testament to the shared humanity that existed beneath the surface, a reminder that the pursuit of authenticity was a journey that was more meaningful when walked together.

One evening, Ava returned to her apartment, surrounded by holographic displays that had come to symbolize her journey. As she gazed at the projections, a holographic message from Sarah appeared before her. "Ava, our connections are a testament to the strength that comes from vulnerability. Lean on us, and allow the bonds we've formed to guide you."

Ava smiled, a sense of warmth and belonging washing over her. The bonds she had formed were a reminder that the pursuit of authenticity was a journey that wasn't meant to be walked alone—it was a journey that was enriched by the connections, support, and understanding of those who walked alongside her.

Chapter 17:

Confronting The Past

As Ava's journey toward authenticity continued, she realized that the pursuit went beyond external transformations and interpersonal connections—it required an inner exploration, a confrontation with the past that had shaped her perceptions, beliefs, and emotions. The holographic displays that once projected scenes of unity now served as reminders of the individual narratives that contributed to the collective tapestry.

Ava's holographic communicator buzzed, and a holographic message from Professor Caine appeared. "Ava," the message read, "the journey toward authenticity requires a willingness to confront the past—the memories, experiences, and emotions that have influenced who you are today. Embrace this exploration with courage."

The holographic displays projected scenes of the city, its bustling streets a reflection of the evolving society. Yet, within Ava's heart, echoes of her past resonated—a past that held memories both joyful and painful, memories that had shaped the person she had become.

One evening, Ava found herself in her childhood home—a place that held memories of laughter, warmth, and the support of her family. The holographic projections transformed the space, bringing to life moments of her upbringing. As she walked through the rooms, the echoes of her past reverberated—a reminder of the innocence and wonder that had once defined her perception of the world.

A holographic projection displayed a message from her father, expressing words of love and encouragement. Ava felt a mixture of emotions—gratitude for the foundation her family had provided and a twinge of longing for the simplicity of childhood.

Yet, as Ava continued her exploration, she found herself drawn to the corners of her past that were tinged with sorrow. Memories of loss, of heartache, and of moments that had left unresolved emotions resurfaced. The holographic displays projected scenes of moments she had long tucked away—a reminder that the pursuit of authenticity required the willingness to acknowledge and confront the complexities of her emotions.

One evening, Ava returned to the holographic cafe, a space where she had engaged in conversations that had transformed her understanding of authenticity. As she sat at a corner table, lost in thought, Emma's holographic message appeared before her. "Ava," the message read, "confronting the past can be challenging, but it's a step toward deeper self-understanding. Embrace the unresolved emotions with gentleness and allow them to guide your journey."

Ava nodded, her heart heavy with the emotions that had resurfaced. The pursuit of authenticity was a journey toward wholeness, a journey that required her to face the aspects of herself that she had long avoided.

Days turned into nights, and Ava found herself revisiting pivotal moments of her past—moments that had left scars, moments that had shaped her fears and insecurities. The holographic displays transformed her apartment into a canvas of memories—a tapestry that wove together the fragments of her journey.

One evening, Ava's holographic communicator buzzed, and a message from Sarah appeared before her. "Ava," the message read, "confronting the past is an act of bravery—an act that allows you to release the hold it has on you. Remember that authenticity is about embracing the totality of your experiences."

Ava's hands trembled as she absorbed Sarah's words. The journey toward authenticity was a journey of courage—a journey that required her to unearth the memories that had remained buried.

One day, Ava found herself standing before a holographic projection—a scene from her past that had long haunted her. The holographic display depicted a moment of conflict, a moment where words had been spoken that had wounded her deeply. As she watched the scene unfold, she felt the weight of the unresolved emotions that had lingered.

A holographic projection of herself appeared before her—an image of her younger self caught in the midst of that painful moment. Ava's eyes welled with tears as she addressed her younger self, speaking words of compassion and understanding. "You are not defined by this moment," she whispered, her voice carrying the reassurance she wished she had received back then.

As she watched the holographic projection, a holographic message from Marcus appeared before her. "Ava," his message read, "confronting the past is a step toward healing—the healing that comes from acknowledging your wounds and granting yourself the grace to move forward."

Ava's heart swelled with a mixture of emotions—relief, sadness, and a sense of release. The holographic displays projected scenes of her journey—the moments of growth, the connections she had formed, and the personal struggles she had faced. The past was no longer a burden; it was a part of her story, a part of the journey that had led her to this point.

One evening, Ava returned to her apartment, surrounded by holographic displays that held the memories of her past. As she gazed at the projections, a holographic message from Nikos appeared before her. "Ava," his message read, "confronting the past is an act of reclaiming your authenticity—a step toward embracing the truth of who you are."

Ava smiled through tears, a sense of liberation washing over her. The pursuit of authenticity was not just about embracing the present; it was about acknowledging the past, healing old wounds, and allowing herself to move forward unburdened by unresolved emotions.

Chapter 18:

Facing Opposition

As Ava's journey toward authenticity continued, she encountered a new challenge—the reality that not everyone within Eudaimonia shared her perspective. The holographic displays that once projected scenes of unity now showcased a diversity of viewpoints, highlighting the complexities of a society in transition.

One evening, Ava found herself in the holographic cafe, engaged in a conversation that took an unexpected turn. As she shared her experiences and insights about authenticity, she noticed skeptical gazes and raised eyebrows from some of the citizens. It became evident that not everyone embraced the pursuit of authenticity in the same way she did.

A holographic projection displayed a message from Emma, reflecting her understanding. "Ava," the message read, "not everyone will share your viewpoint, and that's okay. Embrace the diversity of perspectives—it's a reminder that authenticity encompasses a range of beliefs and experiences."

Ava took a deep breath, reminding herself of the importance of open dialogue and understanding. The pursuit of authenticity wasn't just about her own journey; it was about creating a space where differing perspectives could coexist.

Days turned into nights, and as Ava continued to engage in conversations, she encountered opposition and resistance from individuals who viewed authenticity as a threat to the stability of Eudaimonia. Some argued that the pursuit of authenticity could lead to chaos, while others believed that it might undermine the progress that had been achieved.

One evening, Ava found herself in a heated discussion with a fellow citizen named Lucas. "Ava," Lucas said, his voice tinged with skepticism, "your quest for authenticity—it's a risk. It's a risk to the society we've built, a society that thrives on stability and control."

Ava took a moment to gather her thoughts before responding. "Lucas," she said, her voice measured, "authenticity isn't about dismantling what we've achieved. It's about evolving, growing, and creating a space where individuals can embrace their true selves."

Lucas shook his head, his expression unyielding. "But what about the potential for conflict? What about the challenges that arise when people's beliefs clash?"

Ava regarded him with empathy. "Conflict can arise, but it's through dialogue and understanding that we find common ground. Authenticity isn't a path of isolation; it's a path of connection—a path that allows us to engage with differing perspectives in a meaningful way."

The holographic displays projected scenes of tension and engagement—an illustration of the diversity of perspectives that coexisted within Eudaimonia.

Ava's conversations weren't just about sharing her own insights; they were about listening, learning, and finding common ground.

One day, as Ava walked through the holographic displays, a message from Professor Caine appeared before her. "Ava," the message read, "facing opposition is a part of the journey. Embrace the challenges and use them as opportunities for growth and transformation."

Ava nodded, her determination unwavering. The pursuit of authenticity wasn't meant to be an easy path—it was a path that required resilience, empathy, and a willingness to engage with differing viewpoints.

Weeks turned into months, and as Ava continued to engage in conversations, she began to notice a shift. While opposition still existed, there were individuals who were willing to engage in open dialogue, to listen to her experiences, and to share their own concerns. The holographic cafe had become a space where differing perspectives converged—a space where unity emerged not from agreement, but from understanding.

One evening, Ava found herself in conversation with Zoe, a citizen who had initially expressed skepticism. "Ava," Zoe said, her tone thoughtful, "I've been reflecting on our conversations. While I may not fully embrace the pursuit of authenticity, I can appreciate its importance. It's about finding harmony between individual growth and societal stability."

Ava smiled, grateful for the shift in Zoe's perspective. "Zoe, your willingness to engage in dialogue—it's a testament to the power of open conversation. Authenticity isn't about erasing differences; it's about acknowledging them and finding ways to coexist."

Their conversation deepened, and as they exchanged viewpoints, Ava realized that facing opposition had been an opportunity for growth—for herself and for those who questioned her journey. The holographic displays projected scenes of connection and engagement—a reflection of the progress that could emerge from embracing diverse perspectives.

One evening, as Ava walked through the holographic displays, a message from Marcus appeared before her. "Ava," his message read, "opposition challenges us to refine our beliefs, to strengthen our convictions, and to remain open to growth. Embrace the dialogue, for it is a catalyst for understanding."

Ava nodded, reflecting on the journey that had brought her to this point. The pursuit of authenticity wasn't just a personal quest; it was a journey that intersected with the journeys of others—a journey that required the willingness to face opposition with empathy, to engage in dialogue, and to create a space where differing perspectives could be heard.

One evening, Ava returned to her apartment, surrounded by holographic displays that held the scenes of her conversations. As she gazed at the projections, a holographic message from Sarah appeared before her. "Ava," the message read, "facing opposition is a testament to your commitment to authenticity. Allow the challenges to strengthen your resolve and guide you forward."

Ava smiled, a sense of fulfillment washing over her. The holographic displays were no longer just symbols of unity; they were symbols of the collective journey—a journey that encompassed both agreement and disagreement, both progress and challenges.

Chapter 19:

The Inner Struggle

As Ava's journey toward authenticity continued, she found herself facing an unexpected challenge—an inner struggle that tested the very core of her commitment to embracing her true self. The holographic displays that once projected scenes of unity now revealed the complexity of her emotions, highlighting the depth of her ongoing transformation.

One evening, Ava sat alone in her apartment, surrounded by the holographic displays that held the memories of her journey. An uneasiness settled within her—a sense of restlessness that she hadn't anticipated. The pursuit of authenticity had brought her growth and connection, but it had also brought a heightened awareness of the vulnerabilities she carried.

A holographic projection displayed a message from Emma, her mentor and guide. "Ava," the message read, "inner struggles are a natural part of the journey. Embrace them as opportunities for self-discovery and growth."

Ava sighed, acknowledging Emma's wisdom. Yet, despite the reassurance, the inner turmoil persisted—a turmoil that seemed to stem from a fear of judgment, a fear of not measuring up to the expectations of herself and others.

Days turned into nights, and as Ava engaged in conversations and reflections, the inner struggle intensified. She found herself questioning her decisions, her beliefs, and even the authenticity of her pursuit. The holographic displays projected scenes of self-doubt, highlighting the raw emotions she grappled with.

One evening, Ava's holographic communicator buzzed, and a message from Sarah appeared before her. "Ava," the message read, "the inner struggle is a reflection of your growth. It's a reminder that authenticity requires facing both the light and the shadow within you."

Ava stared at the message, her heart heavy with conflicting emotions. The pursuit of authenticity had transformed her understanding of self, but it had also illuminated the aspects of herself that she had long kept hidden.

One day, as Ava walked through the holographic displays, she found herself immersed in a holographic art gallery. The artworks on display depicted a range of emotions—joy, sorrow, doubt, and resilience. As she studied the artworks, a holographic message from Marcus appeared before her. "Ava," his message read, "the inner struggle is a canvas on which you paint the complexities of your journey. Embrace it as an opportunity to confront your own vulnerabilities."

Ava's gaze shifted from the artworks to the holographic projection of herself—the projection that had become a mirror for her own emotions. The inner struggle was not just a challenge; it was a

reflection of her willingness to delve into the depths
of her being.

One evening, Ava found herself in the holographic
cafe, where conversations often delved into the
complexities of the human experience. As she
engaged in dialogue with fellow citizens, she felt a
mixture of connection and isolation—a reminder
that her inner struggle was a unique journey, yet one
that resonated with the struggles of others.

A holographic projection displayed a message from
Nikos, the philosopher from the outside world.
"Ava," his message read, "the inner struggle is the
crucible in which authenticity is forged. Embrace
the process, for it is a testament to your commitment
to self-discovery."

Ava's hands trembled as she regarded the message.
The inner struggle was not a sign of regression; it
was a sign of growth—a growth that required
confronting the aspects of herself that had long been
denied.

One day, Ava stood before a holographic
projection—a depiction of a mirror that reflected her

own image. As she stared at her holographic reflection, a flood of emotions surged within her. The fear, the doubt, and the vulnerability—all were laid bare before her, reflected in the image that gazed back.

A holographic message from Professor Caine appeared before her. "Ava," the message read, "the inner struggle is a rite of passage—a passage that leads to self-discovery and acceptance. Embrace your emotions and allow them to guide your path."

Ava's eyes filled with tears as she absorbed Professor Caine's words. The inner struggle was not a battle to be won; it was a journey to be embraced—a journey that would lead her to a deeper understanding of herself.

One evening, as Ava walked through the holographic displays, a message from Emma appeared before her. "Ava," the message read, "remember that the pursuit of authenticity is not without its moments of challenge. The inner struggle is a reflection of your commitment to growth and transformation."

Ava nodded, her heart filled with determination. The inner struggle was not just a momentary obstacle; it was a part of her journey—a journey that required the courage to confront her vulnerabilities head-on.

One night, as Ava sat alone in her apartment, surrounded by holographic displays, a holographic message from Sarah appeared before her. "Ava," the message read, "embrace the inner struggle as a reminder of your humanity. Allow it to guide you toward a deeper connection with yourself."

Ava closed her eyes, her breath steadying. The inner struggle was not a detour; it was a pathway—a pathway that would lead her to a more profound understanding of authenticity, one that encompassed both strength and vulnerability.

Chapter 20:

Rediscovery Of Purpose

As Ava continued her journey toward authenticity, the inner struggle had tested her resolve and brought her face to face with her vulnerabilities. Yet, amidst the challenges, a subtle shift began to take place within her—a shift that would lead to the rediscovery of her purpose and a profound transformation of her understanding.

One evening, Ava found herself in the holographic art gallery, surrounded by creative expressions that depicted the myriad facets of the human experience. As she studied the artworks, a holographic message from Emma appeared before her. "Ava," the message read, "the moments of challenge are often the catalysts for rediscovering our purpose. Embrace the shifts within you and allow them to guide your path."

Ava's heart resonated with Emma's words. The inner struggle had not been in vain; it had sparked a process of transformation that was leading her toward a deeper connection with herself and her authenticity.

Days turned into nights, and as Ava engaged in conversations and reflections, she began to notice a new sense of clarity emerging. The holographic displays projected scenes of growth and introspection, illustrating the evolution of her understanding.

One evening, Ava found herself in a conversation with Professor Caine, who had been a guiding presence throughout her journey. "Ava," Professor Caine said, his voice gentle yet filled with wisdom, "the journey of authenticity is not just about self-discovery—it's about rediscovering your purpose, your unique contribution to the world."

Ava regarded him with curiosity. "Professor," she asked, "how do I rediscover my purpose? How do I align it with my journey toward authenticity?"

Professor Caine smiled. "Ava, your purpose is a reflection of your passions, your values, and your authentic self. Reflect on what brings you joy, what resonates deeply within you, and how you can use your journey to inspire and uplift others."

Ava nodded, absorbing his guidance. The rediscovery of purpose was not just a destination; it was a process that required introspection, reflection, and a willingness to align her actions with her authentic self.

Weeks turned into months, and as Ava delved into self-reflection, she found herself drawn to the moments that had brought her the greatest sense of fulfillment—the moments of connection, growth, and support. The holographic displays projected scenes of those experiences, reflecting the path she had walked and the impact she had made.

One day, as Ava walked through the holographic displays, she found herself in the holographic cafe—a space that had been a source of connection and dialogue. As she engaged in conversation with fellow citizens, a sense of purpose began to crystallize within her—an understanding that her journey was not just about personal growth, but about inspiring others to embrace their own authenticity.

A holographic projection displayed a message from Marcus, the philosopher from the outside world. "Ava," his message read, "rediscovering your purpose is a journey of alignment—an alignment between your authentic self and the contribution you can make to the world."

Ava smiled, her heart filled with a newfound sense of purpose. The journey toward authenticity was not just a pursuit of self; it was a pursuit of service—an acknowledgment that her transformation had the potential to ripple outward, touching the lives of others.

One evening, as Ava sat in her apartment, surrounded by holographic displays, a holographic message from Sarah appeared before her. "Ava," the message read, "your purpose is a reflection of your journey—the challenges you've faced, the connections you've formed, and the growth you've experienced. Allow it to guide your actions and inspire your path."

Ava closed her eyes, a sense of alignment washing over her. The rediscovery of purpose was not just a destination; it was a journey that was intimately connected with her journey toward authenticity.

Days turned into nights, and as Ava continued to reflect on her purpose, she felt a renewed sense of energy—a fire within her that burned with intention and clarity. The holographic displays projected scenes of determination, illustrating her commitment to using her journey to make a positive impact on the lives of others.

One evening, Ava found herself back in the holographic art gallery, surrounded by creative expressions that told stories of inspiration, resilience, and transformation. As she studied the artworks, a holographic message from Nikos appeared before her. "Ava," his message read, "your purpose is the compass that guides your journey toward authenticity. Allow it to lead you forward."

Ava's heart swelled with gratitude for the guidance she had received—from mentors, fellow citizens, and her own introspection. The rediscovery of purpose was not just a personal realization; it was a revelation that her journey was intricately connected with a higher calling.

One night, as Ava sat alone in her apartment, surrounded by holographic displays, a holographic message from Emma appeared before her. "Ava," the message read, "the rediscovery of purpose is a profound shift—a shift that aligns your journey with a higher intention. Allow it to infuse your actions with meaning and guide you toward a deeper connection with yourself and others."

Ava smiled, her heart full with a sense of alignment and intention. The holographic displays were no longer just symbols of growth; they were symbols of purpose—a purpose that transcended her own journey and reached out to the world beyond.

Chapter 21:

Embracing Imperfections

As Ava's journey toward authenticity evolved, she encountered a new lesson—a lesson in embracing her imperfections as a vital aspect of her true self. The holographic displays that once projected scenes of unity now illuminated the beauty in the raw and unfiltered aspects of humanity.

One evening, Ava found herself in the holographic cafe, engaged in a conversation that explored the theme of imperfection. As she listened to the stories of fellow citizens, she realized that each person had their own vulnerabilities, quirks, and struggles. The holographic displays projected scenes of candid dialogue, highlighting the shared experiences that bound them together.

A holographic projection displayed a message from Emma, reflecting the essence of authenticity. "Ava," the message read, "embracing imperfections is an act of embracing your humanity. It's about acknowledging the aspects of yourself that make you unique and allowing them to shine."

Ava's heart swelled with recognition. The pursuit of authenticity was not about striving for flawlessness; it was about celebrating the totality of her being, flaws and all.

Days turned into nights, and as Ava engaged in conversations and reflections, she began to notice the subtle ways in which her own imperfections had contributed to her growth. The holographic displays projected scenes of vulnerability, illustrating the moments of authenticity that had forged deeper connections with others.

One evening, Ava found herself in a conversation with Professor Caine, discussing the role of imperfections in the journey toward authenticity. "Ava," Professor Caine said, his voice reflective, "imperfections are not weaknesses; they are reminders of our shared humanity. Embrace them as opportunities for growth and connection."

Ava nodded, her understanding deepening. The holographic displays showcased the spectrum of human experiences—the highs and lows, the strengths and vulnerabilities. It was within the imperfections that the true essence of authenticity resided.

Weeks turned into months, and as Ava navigated her journey, she found herself confronting her own imperfections with a newfound sense of compassion. The holographic displays projected scenes of self-acceptance, highlighting her evolving relationship with the aspects of herself she had once deemed flawed.

One day, as Ava walked through the holographic displays, she found herself in the holographic art gallery. The artworks on display depicted scenes of imperfection turned into sources of beauty and strength—symbolic representations of the transformative power of embracing one's true self.

A holographic message from Marcus appeared before her. "Ava," his message read, "imperfections are the threads that weave the tapestry of your authenticity. Embrace them as gifts that contribute to the richness of your journey."

Ava smiled, her heart lightened by the wisdom in Marcus's words. The pursuit of authenticity was not about erasing imperfections; it was about reframing them as integral parts of her story.

One evening, Ava returned to the holographic cafe, where conversations flowed freely and unfiltered. As she shared her own experiences of imperfection, she noticed a shift—a shift in the way others responded. Instead of judgment, she encountered understanding and empathy, illustrating the power of vulnerability to bridge the gaps between individuals.

A holographic projection displayed a message from Nikos, the philosopher from the outside world. "Ava," his message read, "embracing imperfections is a practice in self-compassion. It's a journey that allows you to stand fully in your truth and connect with others on a deeper level."

Ava's gaze turned to the holographic displays that projected scenes of authenticity—the moments of imperfection that had given rise to growth and connection. The imperfections were not obstacles to be overcome; they were stepping stones toward a more genuine understanding of herself.

One day, Ava stood before a holographic projection—a depiction of a mirror that reflected her image, imperfections and all. As she stared at her holographic reflection, a wave of acceptance washed over her. The holographic projection displayed a message from Sarah. "Ava," the message read, "your imperfections are not blemishes; they are brushstrokes that add depth to your canvas. Embrace them as unique facets of your journey."

Ava's eyes filled with tears as she regarded the message. The pursuit of authenticity was not just about the external journey—it was about the internal journey of self-acceptance and self-love.

One evening, as Ava sat alone in her apartment, surrounded by holographic displays, a holographic message from Emma appeared before her. "Ava," the message read, "embrace your imperfections with

gratitude, for they are the portals through which
your authenticity shines. Allow them to guide you
toward a deeper connection with yourself and
others."

Ava smiled through tears, a sense of liberation
enveloping her. The holographic displays were no
longer just symbols of growth and transformation;
they were symbols of self-love and acceptance—a
celebration of her journey, imperfections and all.

Chapter 22:

The Inner Circle

As Ava's journey toward authenticity continued, she found herself drawn into a new dimension of connection—a circle of individuals who shared her commitment to embracing their true selves. The holographic displays that once projected scenes of unity now showcased the power of community in amplifying personal growth.

One evening, Ava received an invitation to a gathering of like-minded individuals who had been following her journey. As she entered the holographic space, she was greeted by warm smiles and open arms. The holographic displays projected scenes of camaraderie and shared purpose, highlighting the sense of belonging that she had found.

A holographic projection displayed a message from Emma, acknowledging the significance of community. "Ava," the message read, "the journey toward authenticity is not meant to be solitary. Embrace the connections you form and allow them to support your growth."

Ava's heart swelled with gratitude as she regarded the message. The pursuit of authenticity was not just an individual endeavor; it was a collective journey that gained strength from the support of others.

Days turned into nights, and as Ava engaged in conversations and shared experiences with her newfound community, she realized the power of the connections she had formed. The holographic displays projected scenes of shared stories and shared challenges, illustrating the sense of kinship that had emerged.

One evening, Ava found herself in a conversation with Professor Caine, reflecting on the significance of the inner circle. "Ava," Professor Caine said, his voice resonant with wisdom, "the inner circle is a reflection of the bonds you've formed—a reflection of the community that uplifts you and walks alongside you."

Ava nodded, her heart filled with appreciation for the connections that had blossomed from her journey. The holographic displays showcased the diversity of experiences and backgrounds within the inner circle—a diversity that enriched the collective wisdom.

Weeks turned into months, and as Ava spent time with her inner circle, she found herself inspired by the stories of growth and transformation shared by others. The holographic displays projected scenes of mutual support, highlighting the way each individual contributed to the shared journey.

One day, as Ava walked through the holographic displays, she found herself immersed in a holographic garden—a symbol of the blossoming connections she had cultivated. As she engaged in conversation with fellow members of her inner circle, she realized that they were not just allies on her journey; they were friends who celebrated her victories and stood by her side during challenges.

A holographic message from Marcus appeared before her. "Ava," his message read, "the inner circle is a space where authenticity thrives. It's a space where your growth is mirrored and celebrated by others who walk a similar path."

Ava smiled, her heart warmed by the sentiment in Marcus's words. The pursuit of authenticity was not just about personal transformation; it was about fostering a sense of belonging and mutual encouragement.

One evening, Ava returned to the holographic cafe—a space where connections had been formed and ideas had been shared. As she engaged in conversation with her inner circle, she noticed a deep sense of resonance in their discussions—a resonance that stemmed from their shared commitment to authenticity.

A holographic projection displayed a message from Nikos, the philosopher from the outside world. "Ava," his message read, "the inner circle is a reflection of your journey's impact on others. Embrace the connections you've forged and allow them to guide your path."

Ava's gaze turned to the holographic displays that projected scenes of unity—the moments of shared laughter, shared reflections, and shared growth. The inner circle was not just a support system; it was a reminder of the collective potential to create a more authentic and connected world.

One day, Ava stood before a holographic projection—a depiction of interconnected circles that represented her inner circle and its influence on her journey. As she gazed at the holographic image, a holographic message from Sarah appeared before her. "Ava," the message read, "the inner circle is a testament to your courage and vulnerability. It's a circle that amplifies your authenticity and inspires others to embrace their own journeys."

Ava's eyes welled with tears as she absorbed Sarah's words. The inner circle was not just a group of individuals; it was a symbol of the ripple effect that authenticity could create—a ripple that extended far beyond the individual, reaching into the lives of others.

One evening, as Ava sat alone in her apartment, surrounded by holographic displays, a holographic message from Emma appeared before her. "Ava," the message read, "cherish the connections you've formed within the inner circle. Allow them to remind you that the pursuit of authenticity is a collective endeavor that transforms not only individuals, but also the fabric of society."

Ava smiled, a profound sense of gratitude washing over her. The holographic displays were no longer just symbols of growth and connection; they were symbols of community—a community that stood by her side and lifted her spirit as she continued her journey toward authenticity.

Chapter 23:

Facing The Truth

As Ava's journey toward authenticity continued to unfold, she encountered a moment that would test the very foundation of her understanding. The holographic displays that once projected scenes of growth and unity now revealed a truth that would require her to question her beliefs and confront her own biases.

One evening, Ava found herself in a holographic auditorium, attending a lecture on the history of Eudaimonia. The holographic screens displayed scenes from the past—a past that had been carefully curated to present a harmonious narrative of progress and unity.

However, as the lecture continued, Ava's intuition started to prick at her. Something about the version of history being presented didn't quite align with the diverse perspectives she had encountered on her journey. The holographic displays projected scenes of the lecture, illustrating Ava's growing unease.

A holographic projection displayed a message from Emma, a reminder to trust her instincts. "Ava," the message read, "authenticity requires the courage to question what seems to be, to uncover the layers of truth that lie beneath the surface."

Ava's heart raced as she considered Emma's words. The pursuit of authenticity was not just about embracing her own truth; it was about seeking truth in the world around her.

Days turned into nights, and as Ava engaged in conversations and reflections, she began to delve deeper into the history of Eudaimonia. She sought out hidden archives and spoke to citizens who had experienced the society's evolution firsthand. The holographic displays projected scenes of research and exploration, capturing Ava's determination to uncover the truth.

One evening, Ava found herself in a conversation with Professor Caine, discussing the importance of facing uncomfortable truths. "Ava," Professor Caine said, his voice somber yet resolute, "confronting the truth is a courageous act—one that challenges our perceptions and invites us to evolve."

Ava nodded, her understanding deepening. The holographic displays showcased the complexity of truth—the layers that were often concealed by the narratives constructed by society.

Weeks turned into months, and as Ava continued her investigation, she uncovered discrepancies and contradictions in the official history of Eudaimonia. The holographic displays projected scenes of revelation, illustrating her growing awareness of a truth that had been obscured by the veneer of perfection.

One day, as Ava walked through the holographic displays, she found herself in a virtual archive—a repository of documents and recordings from the past. As she sifted through the materials, she stumbled upon a holographic message from Marcus. "Ava," his message read, "facing the truth requires us to dismantle the illusions we've constructed. Embrace the discomfort, for it is a catalyst for growth."

Ava's hands trembled as she absorbed Marcus's message. The pursuit of authenticity was not a journey of convenience; it was a journey of uncovering truths that had been hidden from view.

One evening, Ava returned to her apartment, surrounded by holographic displays that held the evidence of her investigation. As she reviewed the materials, a holographic message from Sarah appeared before her. "Ava," the message read, "facing the truth is not just about seeking external truths—it's about confronting the truths within yourself, the biases and assumptions that shape your perspective."

Ava closed her eyes, her thoughts turning inward. The pursuit of authenticity required self-awareness—a willingness to confront her own preconceived notions and biases.

One day, Ava stood before a holographic projection—a depiction of shattered illusions and unveiled truths. As she stared at the holographic image, a holographic message from Nikos appeared before her. "Ava," his message read, "the truth may be uncomfortable, but it is a doorway to a deeper understanding of reality. Embrace it as a catalyst for transformation."

Ava's gaze turned to the holographic displays that projected scenes of revelation—the moments of truth that had reshaped her perception of the world around her. The pursuit of authenticity was not just a path of self-discovery; it was a path of uncovering the hidden layers of reality.

One evening, as Ava sat alone in her apartment, surrounded by holographic displays, a holographic message from Emma appeared before her. "Ava," the message read, "facing the truth is a pivotal moment in your journey. Allow it to guide you toward a more authentic understanding of yourself and the world."

Ava took a deep breath, a sense of resolve filling her. The holographic displays were no longer just symbols of growth and unity; they were symbols of truth—a truth that demanded her attention and compelled her to reevaluate her beliefs.

Chapter 24:

A Difficult Choice

As Ava's journey toward authenticity led her deeper into the layers of truth, she encountered a crossroads—a difficult choice that would test the very essence of her commitment. The holographic displays that once projected scenes of growth and unity now revealed the weight of a decision that could shape her future in Eudaimonia.

One evening, Ava found herself standing before a holographic projection—a depiction of two diverging paths. One path was marked by her authenticity, a journey of embracing her true self and confronting uncomfortable truths. The other path represented the familiar route of conformity, following the societal expectations of Eudaimonia.

Ava's heart ached as she regarded the holographic image. The pursuit of authenticity had brought her wisdom, growth, and connection, but it had also placed her in a position where she had to choose between personal integrity and societal harmony.

A holographic projection displayed a message from Emma, a reminder that choices define our journey. "Ava," the message read, "every choice you make shapes your authenticity. Choose with the knowledge that your path holds the potential to inspire change."

Ava's thoughts were a whirlwind of conflicting emotions. The pursuit of authenticity was not just about her personal growth; it was about the impact she could have on the society she had grown up in.

Days turned into nights, and as Ava deliberated her decision, she sought counsel from her inner circle. The holographic displays projected scenes of heartfelt conversations, illustrating the range of perspectives that surrounded her.

One evening, Ava found herself in a conversation with Professor Caine, who listened to her doubts and uncertainties with compassion. "Ava," Professor Caine said, his voice filled with empathy, "difficult choices are often mirrors that reflect our values and priorities. Consider the long-term implications of your decision."

Ava nodded, absorbing his wisdom. The holographic displays showcased the significance of her choice—a choice that extended beyond her individual journey.

Weeks turned into months, and as Ava contemplated her decision, she found herself torn between the pull of authenticity and the familiarity of conformity. The holographic displays projected scenes of inner turmoil, capturing her struggle to align her choices with her values.

One day, as Ava walked through the holographic displays, she found herself in a holographic garden—a symbol of growth and transformation. As she wandered among the holographic flowers, a holographic message from Marcus appeared before her. "Ava," his message read, "a difficult choice is a canvas on which you paint the hues of your authenticity. Embrace the challenge, for it is a testament to your commitment to truth."

Ava's thoughts lingered on Marcus's message. The pursuit of authenticity was not without its challenges; it was a journey that required her to make choices that resonated with the depths of her being.

One evening, Ava returned to her apartment, surrounded by holographic displays that held memories of her journey. As she gazed at the holographic images, a holographic message from Sarah appeared before her. "Ava," the message read, "remember that your choices are the threads that weave the fabric of your story. Choose with integrity and let your authenticity shine."

Ava closed her eyes, her thoughts turning inward. The pursuit of authenticity was not just about external growth; it was about staying true to herself, even in the face of difficult decisions.

One day, Ava stood before the holographic projection—a depiction of the crossroads she faced. As she stared at the holographic image, a holographic message from Nikos appeared before her. "Ava," his message read, "a difficult choice is an opportunity to embody your authenticity. Trust the voice within you and choose the path that aligns with your true self."

Ava's gaze shifted between the two paths—the one of authenticity and the one of conformity. The choice was before her, a choice that carried the weight of her values and her vision of a more authentic Eudaimonia.

One evening, as Ava sat alone in her apartment, surrounded by holographic displays, a holographic message from Emma appeared before her. "Ava," the message read, "difficult choices are the crucibles in which our authenticity is forged. Allow your heart to guide you toward a decision that aligns with your purpose and values."

Ava took a deep breath, her heart steadying. The holographic displays were no longer just symbols of growth and connection; they were symbols of choice—a choice that would define her journey toward authenticity.

Chapter 25:

Reckoning With Eudaimonia

As Ava's journey toward authenticity reached a
pivotal juncture, she found herself facing a
reckoning—a confrontation with the very society
she had known. The holographic displays that once
projected scenes of unity and progress now revealed
the consequences of her choices and the complexity
of challenging the status quo.

One evening, Ava stood before the entrance to the
Eudaimonia Council—a symbol of authority and
governance. Her heart pounded as she prepared to
address the council members, including those who
had upheld the illusions that had been shattered by
her pursuit of authenticity. The holographic displays
projected scenes of tension and anticipation,
capturing the gravity of the moment.

Ava's journey had brought her to this point—a point
of no return where her commitment to authenticity

clashed with the expectations of Eudaimonia. She took a deep breath, drawing on the strength she had gained from her inner circle and her own transformation.

A holographic projection displayed a message from Emma, a reminder to stand firm in her truth. "Ava," the message read, "the reckoning is a culmination of your journey—a moment of truth where you hold the mirror to the society you seek to change."

Ava's thoughts were a maelstrom of emotions as she considered Emma's words. The pursuit of authenticity was not just a personal endeavor; it was a catalyst for change that had the potential to reverberate throughout Eudaimonia.

Days turned into nights, and as Ava prepared to address the council, she sought counsel from her inner circle. The holographic displays projected scenes of support and camaraderie, illustrating the strength she drew from her connections.

One evening, Ava found herself in a conversation with Professor Caine, who offered guidance on navigating the reckoning. "Ava," Professor Caine said, his voice steady, "the reckoning is a confrontation between the individual and the collective. Trust in your journey and speak from the depths of your authenticity."

Ava nodded, absorbing his wisdom. The holographic displays showcased the significance of her presence—the potential to disrupt the narratives that had kept Eudaimonia in a state of complacency.

Weeks turned into months, and as Ava contemplated her address to the council, she found herself grappling with the consequences of her choices. The holographic displays projected scenes of inner reflection, capturing her struggle to reconcile her commitment to authenticity with the potential fallout of her actions.

One day, as Ava walked through the holographic displays, she found herself in a virtual square—a space where citizens gathered for important announcements and discussions. As she stood in the square, a holographic message from Marcus appeared before her. "Ava," his message read, "the reckoning is a pivotal moment that demands courage. Allow your truth to be a beacon that guides the way."

Ava's gaze turned to the holographic displays that projected scenes of public discourse—the moments where the status quo had been questioned and change had been ignited. The reckoning was not just about her; it was about a collective shift toward a more authentic Eudaimonia.

One evening, Ava returned to her apartment, surrounded by holographic displays that held memories of her journey. As she contemplated the consequences of her impending reckoning, a holographic message from Sarah appeared before her. "Ava," the message read, "the reckoning is a mirror that reflects the transformation you've undergone. Embrace it as an opportunity to catalyze change."

Ava closed her eyes, her thoughts turning inward. The pursuit of authenticity was not just a personal journey; it was a journey that had the potential to alter the trajectory of Eudaimonia itself.

One day, Ava stood before the holographic projection—a depiction of the council chamber and the council members who held the power to shape the society's future. As she prepared to address them, a holographic message from Nikos appeared before her. "Ava," his message read, "the reckoning is a bridge between the old and the new. Stand tall and speak your truth with conviction."

Ava's gaze shifted between the holographic images—the council chamber and the paths that had led her to this moment. The reckoning was not just about the choices before her; it was about the choices she was offering to the society she had grown up in.

One evening, as Ava sat alone in her apartment, surrounded by holographic displays, a holographic message from Emma appeared before her. "Ava," the message read, "the reckoning is a testament to your journey—a journey of authenticity, transformation, and courage. Allow it to shape not only your path, but also the path of Eudaimonia."

Ava took a deep breath, a sense of purpose filling her. The holographic displays were no longer just symbols of growth and unity; they were symbols of reckoning—a reckoning that demanded her truth and offered the potential for a more authentic and inclusive society.

Chapter 26:

Seeds of Revolution

As Ava faced the council of Eudaimonia and shared her truth, she could feel the weight of her words reverberate through the chamber. The holographic displays that once projected scenes of harmony and progress now showcased the pivotal moment where seeds of revolution were sown.

Ava's voice resonated with unwavering conviction as she addressed the council members, recounting her journey of authenticity and the truths she had uncovered. The holographic displays projected scenes of rapt attention and contemplation among the council members, capturing the magnitude of her impact.

The reckoning had arrived—a reckoning that would shape the course of Eudaimonia's future. As Ava spoke, her words cut through the illusions that had been carefully constructed, illuminating the hidden layers of truth that lay beneath.

A holographic projection displayed a message from Emma, a reminder that truth has the power to ignite change. "Ava," the message read, "the seeds of revolution are sown when authenticity challenges the foundations of the status quo. Let your words be a catalyst for transformation."

Ava's heart raced as she considered Emma's words. The pursuit of authenticity was not just an individual journey; it was a movement that had the potential to awaken a society from its slumber.

Days turned into nights, and as Ava's address to the council spread throughout Eudaimonia, she became a symbol of courage and change. The holographic displays projected scenes of citizens engaged in discussions, questioning the narratives they had accepted for so long.

One evening, Ava found herself in a conversation with Professor Caine, reflecting on the power of her words. "Ava," Professor Caine said, his voice filled with hope, "the seeds of revolution take root when truth resonates with the hearts of many. Your journey has ignited a spark that has the potential to light a path toward a more authentic society."

Ava nodded, absorbing his insight. The holographic displays showcased the collective response to her reckoning—the emergence of a shared vision for change.

Weeks turned into months, and as citizens engaged in dialogues inspired by Ava's reckoning, a movement for authenticity began to take shape. The holographic displays projected scenes of gatherings, discussions, and the sharing of personal stories, illustrating the way individuals were banding together to challenge the norms of Eudaimonia.

One day, as Ava walked through the holographic displays, she found herself in the midst of a holographic protest—a manifestation of the movement that had been sparked by her words. The holographic signs held messages of unity, authenticity, and transformation. As she joined her fellow citizens, Ava could feel the collective energy of change swirling around her.

A holographic message from Marcus appeared before her. "Ava," his message read, "seeds of revolution grow when individuals recognize their power to shape their reality. Embrace the momentum you've ignited and continue to lead with authenticity."

Ava's heart swelled with gratitude as she regarded Marcus's message. The pursuit of authenticity was not just about her journey; it was about inspiring others to step into their own truth and drive change.

One evening, Ava returned to the holographic cafe—a space that had witnessed her growth and transformation. As she engaged in conversation with fellow citizens, she noticed a renewed sense of purpose and determination in their voices. The holographic displays showcased the unity and solidarity that had emerged from the movement for authenticity.

A holographic projection displayed a message from Nikos, the philosopher from the outside world. "Ava," his message read, "seeds of revolution flourish when individuals choose to embody their values. Your journey has sparked a fire that has the potential to reshape the very fabric of Eudaimonia."

Ava's gaze turned to the holographic displays that projected scenes of action and transformation—the moments where individuals had risen up to challenge the norms and expectations that had held them captive for so long. The movement was not just about her; it was about a collective striving for a more authentic and inclusive society.

One day, Ava stood before a holographic projection—a depiction of the movement for authenticity spreading like wildfire throughout Eudaimonia. As she stared at the holographic image, a holographic message from Sarah appeared before her. "Ava," the message read, "the seeds of revolution are a testament to your courage and tenacity. Nurture them with authenticity and watch as they blossom into lasting change."

Ava's eyes filled with tears as she absorbed Sarah's words. The holographic displays were no longer just symbols of growth and connection; they were symbols of revolution—a revolution fueled by

authenticity and driven by individuals who were no
longer willing to accept the status quo.

One evening, as Ava sat alone in her apartment,
surrounded by holographic displays, a holographic
message from Emma appeared before her. "Ava,"
the message read, "the seeds of revolution are the
legacy of your journey—a legacy that transcends the
individual and shapes the destiny of Eudaimonia."

Ava smiled, a profound sense of purpose filling her.
The holographic displays were no longer just
symbols of her personal transformation; they were
symbols of a movement—a movement that had the
power to reshape Eudaimonia and inspire a new era
of authenticity.

Chapter 27:

Facing Opposition

As the movement for authenticity gained momentum within Eudaimonia, Ava found herself facing a new challenge—opposition from those who were invested in preserving the existing order. The holographic displays that once projected scenes of unity and change now revealed the complexities of challenging deeply ingrained beliefs.

One evening, Ava stood before a holographic gathering—a congregation of citizens who had aligned themselves with the traditional ideals of Eudaimonia. The holographic displays projected scenes of tension and division, capturing the clash between the emerging movement and those who resisted change.

Ava's determination was unwavering as she addressed the gathering, advocating for a more inclusive and authentic society. The holographic displays showcased the varying reactions of the audience—some listening with open minds, while others displayed skepticism and resistance.

The opposition had materialized—a counterforce to the movement she had ignited. As Ava spoke, she could feel the weight of her words against the currents of resistance that had been set in motion.

A holographic projection displayed a message from Emma, a reminder that change is often met with opposition. "Ava," the message read, "facing opposition is a testament to the impact of your movement. Stay true to your values and allow your authenticity to guide your response."

Ava's thoughts were a maelstrom of emotions as she considered Emma's words. The pursuit of authenticity was not just about advocating for change; it was about navigating the challenges that arose in the face of opposition.

Days turned into nights, and as the movement encountered resistance, Ava sought counsel from her inner circle. The holographic displays projected scenes of discussions and strategy sessions, illustrating the collaborative efforts of those who were aligned with the vision of a more authentic Eudaimonia.

One evening, Ava found herself in a conversation with Professor Caine, reflecting on the nature of opposition. "Ava," Professor Caine said, his voice calm yet resolute, "opposition arises when the established order feels threatened. Stay committed to your vision, and remember that change often requires patience and perseverance."

Ava nodded, absorbing his wisdom. The holographic displays showcased the diversity of perspectives within Eudaimonia—a diversity that mirrored the complexity of the societal transformation she sought to bring about.

Weeks turned into months, and as opposition continued to challenge the movement, Ava realized that her journey was evolving. The holographic displays projected scenes of resilience and determination, capturing her ongoing commitment to navigating the obstacles that arose.

One day, as Ava walked through the holographic displays, she found herself in a virtual square—a space where citizens voiced their concerns and disagreements. As she listened to the varying perspectives, a holographic message from Marcus appeared before her. "Ava," his message read, "facing opposition is an opportunity to engage in dialogue and bridge divides. Embrace the challenge of finding common ground."

Ava's gaze turned to the holographic displays that projected scenes of heated discussions—the moments where opposing viewpoints clashed and collided. The opposition was not just an obstacle; it was a chance to foster understanding and empathy.

One evening, Ava returned to her apartment, surrounded by holographic displays that held memories of her journey. As she reflected on the challenges posed by opposition, a holographic message from Sarah appeared before her. "Ava," the message read, "facing opposition requires strength and compassion. Stay true to your authenticity and approach disagreements with an open heart."

Ava closed her eyes, her thoughts turning inward. The pursuit of authenticity was not just about advocating for change; it was about demonstrating the transformative power of authentic dialogue in the face of opposition.

One day, Ava stood before a holographic projection—a depiction of the opposing forces within Eudaimonia. As she contemplated the division that existed, a holographic message from Nikos appeared before her. "Ava," his message read, "opposition is a reflection of the diversity within a society. Embrace the challenge of fostering unity amid differing perspectives."

Ava's gaze shifted between the holographic images—the division that was visible and the unity that could be cultivated. The opposition was not just a barrier; it was an invitation to bridge divides and create a more authentic and connected society.

One evening, as Ava sat alone in her apartment, surrounded by holographic displays, a holographic message from Emma appeared before her. "Ava," the message read, "facing opposition is a testament to the resilience of your movement. Allow it to remind you of the transformative power of authenticity in breaking down barriers."

Ava took a deep breath, a renewed sense of purpose filling her. The holographic displays were no longer just symbols of growth and unity; they were symbols of opposition—a challenge that had the potential to strengthen the movement and create a more inclusive Eudaimonia.

Chapter 28:

A New Vision

As Ava confronted the opposition that had arisen in response to the movement for authenticity, she recognized the need to evolve her approach. The holographic displays that once projected scenes of unity and growth now revealed the complexity of unifying a society divided by differing viewpoints.

One evening, Ava found herself standing in a holographic square—a space that had witnessed both unity and discord. Citizens from various perspectives had gathered, their holographic signs expressing divergent opinions on the direction of Eudaimonia. The holographic displays projected scenes of tension and uncertainty, capturing the challenge of fostering understanding amid disagreement.

Ava's determination remained unwavering as she addressed the gathering, acknowledging the differences that existed while emphasizing the shared humanity that united them. The holographic displays showcased the varying reactions of the audience—some nodding in agreement, others still guarded and skeptical.

A new vision was emerging—an aspiration for a more inclusive Eudaimonia that transcended the barriers that had arisen. As Ava spoke, she sought to bridge divides and ignite a sense of common purpose.

A holographic projection displayed a message from Emma, a reminder that a new vision requires empathy and compassion. "Ava," the message read, "crafting a new vision is a testament to the depth of your commitment. Envision a future that encompasses the aspirations of all citizens."

Ava's thoughts were a whirlwind of possibilities as she considered Emma's words. The pursuit of authenticity was not just about challenging the norms; it was about creating a space where differing perspectives could coexist in harmony.

Days turned into nights, and as Ava continued to navigate the complexities of division, she sought counsel from her inner circle. The holographic displays projected scenes of conversations and brainstorming sessions, illustrating the collective effort to formulate a vision that would resonate with all citizens.

One evening, Ava found herself in a conversation with Professor Caine, reflecting on the challenges of unifying a divided society. "Ava," Professor Caine said, his voice reflective, "a new vision emerges when individuals find common ground amid differences. Stay focused on the values that unite humanity and inspire change."

Ava nodded, absorbing his wisdom. The holographic displays showcased the importance of empathy—the ability to see beyond opposing viewpoints and recognize the shared aspirations of Eudaimonia's citizens.

Weeks turned into months, and as Ava worked to articulate a new vision, she realized that her journey had evolved once again. The holographic displays projected scenes of collaboration and creativity, capturing the collective effort to envision a society that honored authenticity and diversity.

One day, as Ava walked through the holographic displays, she found herself in a virtual park—a symbol of harmony and tranquility. As she strolled among the holographic trees, a holographic message from Marcus appeared before her. "Ava," his message read, "a new vision requires you to transcend divisions and inspire unity. Embrace the challenge of crafting a narrative that resonates with the hearts of all citizens."

Ava's gaze turned to the holographic displays that projected scenes of dialogue and discourse—the moments where individuals from different walks of life engaged in conversations that challenged assumptions and fostered understanding. The new vision was not just about her; it was about cultivating a shared narrative that honored the richness of diversity.

One evening, Ava returned to her apartment, surrounded by holographic displays that held memories of her journey. As she reflected on the complexities of unifying a divided society, a holographic message from Sarah appeared before her. "Ava," the message read, "a new vision is a bridge that connects differing perspectives. Stay true to your authenticity and invite citizens to envision a future that reflects their values."

Ava closed her eyes, her thoughts turning inward. The pursuit of authenticity was not just about advocating for change; it was about inviting individuals to contribute to a vision that encompassed the essence of their aspirations.

One day, Ava stood before a holographic projection—a depiction of the diverse citizens of Eudaimonia engaging in conversations about the new vision. As she contemplated the unity that was emerging, a holographic message from Nikos appeared before her. "Ava," his message read, "a new vision emerges when individuals recognize their interconnectedness. Lead with humility and empower citizens to be architects of their collective future."

Ava's gaze shifted between the holographic images—the diversity that was visible and the unity that was being nurtured. The new vision was not just an aspiration; it was a testament to the potential for change when individuals come together with shared purpose.

One evening, as Ava sat alone in her apartment, surrounded by holographic displays, a holographic message from Emma appeared before her. "Ava," the message read, "a new vision is a reflection of your growth and evolution. Allow it to transcend the divisions and inspire a future that honors authenticity and unity."

Ava smiled, a renewed sense of determination filling her. The holographic displays were no longer just symbols of growth and transformation; they were symbols of a new vision—a vision that had the power to reshape Eudaimonia and guide its citizens toward a more inclusive and authentic future.

Chapter 29:

Reconciliation

As Ava continued to navigate the challenges of unifying a divided society, she recognized the need for reconciliation—a process that would bridge the gaps between the various factions within Eudaimonia. The holographic displays that once projected scenes of division now revealed the potential for healing and transformation.

One evening, Ava found herself standing in the heart of the city—a symbolic gathering place for citizens who held differing perspectives. The holographic displays projected scenes of citizens from different walks of life, their holographic signs representing the diversity of opinions that existed.

Ava's determination to foster reconciliation was evident as she addressed the gathering, inviting individuals to engage in constructive conversations that could lead to understanding and unity. The holographic displays showcased the mixed reactions of the audience—some expressing openness, while others remained guarded.

The process of reconciliation had begun—a journey that required patience, empathy, and a commitment to finding common ground. As Ava spoke, she encouraged individuals to recognize their shared humanity and the potential for collaboration.

A holographic projection displayed a message from Emma, a reminder that reconciliation is born from the willingness to listen and empathize. "Ava," the message read, "the path of reconciliation is a testament to your leadership. Guide individuals toward a shared vision that reflects their aspirations."

Ava's thoughts were a mix of hope and determination as she considered Emma's words. The pursuit of authenticity was not just about advocating for change; it was about fostering a sense of belonging and understanding among all citizens.

Days turned into nights, and as Ava embarked on the journey of reconciliation, she sought counsel from her inner circle. The holographic displays projected scenes of conversations and dialogues, illustrating the effort to create spaces where individuals could engage in constructive exchanges.

One evening, Ava found herself in a conversation with Professor Caine, reflecting on the challenges of reconciling differing perspectives. "Ava," Professor Caine said, his voice filled with wisdom, "reconciliation is a testament to the power of empathy. Lead by example and demonstrate the transformative potential of understanding."

Ava nodded, absorbing his guidance. The holographic displays showcased the importance of creating safe spaces for individuals to share their stories, challenges, and hopes for Eudaimonia's future.

Weeks turned into months, and as Ava facilitated dialogues between different factions, she began to witness the seeds of reconciliation taking root. The holographic displays projected scenes of individuals from opposing viewpoints engaging in respectful conversations, gradually building bridges of understanding.

One day, as Ava walked through the holographic displays, she found herself in a virtual garden—a representation of growth and harmony. As she observed individuals sharing their experiences and listening to one another, a holographic message from Marcus appeared before her. "Ava," his message read, "reconciliation is a journey of transformation for both individuals and society. Embrace the challenge of nurturing unity and understanding."

Ava's gaze turned to the holographic displays that projected scenes of healing conversations—the moments where individuals set aside their differences and engaged in authentic interactions. The process of reconciliation was not just about reaching an agreement; it was about fostering a sense of community and shared purpose.

One evening, Ava returned to her apartment, surrounded by holographic displays that held memories of her journey. As she reflected on the progress of reconciliation, a holographic message from Sarah appeared before her. "Ava," the message read, "reconciliation requires patience and compassion. Stay true to your authenticity and guide citizens toward a vision that honors their individuality while embracing unity."

Ava closed her eyes, her thoughts turning inward. The pursuit of authenticity was not just about advocating for change; it was about facilitating a space where individuals could come together in pursuit of a better society.

One day, Ava stood before a holographic projection—a depiction of individuals from different factions engaging in a dialogue of reconciliation. As she contemplated the unity that was emerging, a holographic message from Nikos appeared before her. "Ava," his message read, "reconciliation is a reflection of the collective desire for growth and transformation. Lead with humility and guide citizens toward a future that values diversity and unity."

Ava's gaze shifted between the holographic images—the division that was visible and the unity that was being nurtured. Reconciliation was not just

an ideal; it was a tangible process that had the power
to shape the destiny of Eudaimonia.

One evening, as Ava sat alone in her apartment,
surrounded by holographic displays, a holographic
message from Emma appeared before her. "Ava,"
the message read, "reconciliation is a testament to
your commitment to change. Allow it to remind you
of the transformative power of authentic dialogue in
fostering unity."

Ava smiled, a profound sense of purpose filling her.
The holographic displays were no longer just
symbols of growth and unity; they were symbols of
reconciliation—a reconciliation that had the
potential to reshape Eudaimonia and lead its citizens
toward a more harmonious and inclusive future.

Chapter 30:

A Balanced Eudaimonia

As Ava's journey of transformation and reconciliation continued, she found herself on the brink of a new era for Eudaimonia—one marked by balance, authenticity, and unity. The holographic displays that once projected scenes of division and dissent now showcased the culmination of her efforts and the birth of a more harmonious society.

One evening, Ava stood before a holographic gathering—a representation of the diverse citizens of Eudaimonia who had come together in pursuit of a shared vision. The holographic displays projected scenes of individuals from different walks of life, their holographic signs now bearing messages of unity and hope.

Ava's voice resonated with a profound sense of purpose as she addressed the gathering, announcing the collective achievement of reconciliation and the formulation of a new vision for Eudaimonia. The holographic displays showcased scenes of anticipation and excitement, capturing the transformative power of unity and collaboration.

A new chapter had begun—an era defined by a balanced Eudaimonia that honored authenticity and diversity. As Ava spoke, she invited citizens to participate in shaping the society's future and to embrace a more inclusive and harmonious way of life.

A holographic projection displayed a message from Emma, a reminder that a balanced society is one where all voices are valued. "Ava," the message read, "the establishment of a balanced Eudaimonia is a testament to your leadership. Continue to guide individuals toward a future that reflects their shared values."

Ava's thoughts were a mix of fulfillment and humility as she considered Emma's words. The pursuit of authenticity was not just about advocating for change; it was about creating a space where every citizen could contribute to a brighter future.

Days turned into nights, and as Ava worked alongside her inner circle and citizens of Eudaimonia, the vision of a balanced society began to take shape. The holographic displays projected scenes of collaboration, innovation, and a shared commitment to embracing diversity and authenticity.

One evening, Ava found herself in a conversation with Professor Caine, reflecting on the significance of establishing a balanced Eudaimonia. "Ava," Professor Caine said, his voice imbued with hope, "a balanced society arises when individuals recognize their interconnectedness and embrace their unique contributions. Your journey has paved the way for a future where authenticity and unity coexist."

Ava nodded, absorbing his insights. The holographic displays showcased the richness of perspectives within Eudaimonia—a richness that now contributed to the tapestry of a more balanced and authentic society.

Weeks turned into months, and as citizens embraced the vision of a balanced Eudaimonia, Ava witnessed

the transformation of her society. The holographic
displays projected scenes of cooperation, shared
initiatives, and a sense of shared purpose that
transcended past divisions.

One day, as Ava walked through the holographic
displays, she found herself in a virtual park—a place
of unity and harmony. As she observed individuals
engaging in discussions and collaborative projects, a
holographic message from Marcus appeared before
her. "Ava," his message read, "a balanced society
flourishes when individuals are empowered to
contribute their unique strengths. Nurture the unity
that has emerged and continue to inspire a future
that values authenticity."

Ava's gaze turned to the holographic displays that
projected scenes of individuals working together—
the moments where differences were celebrated and
contributions were recognized. The balanced
Eudaimonia was not just a concept; it was a reality
that had been shaped by the collective efforts of its
citizens.

One evening, Ava returned to her apartment,
surrounded by holographic displays that held

memories of her journey. As she reflected on the establishment of a balanced Eudaimonia, a holographic message from Sarah appeared before her. "Ava," the message read, "a balanced society is a testament to your resilience and commitment. Stay true to your authenticity and guide citizens toward a future that honors their individuality while nurturing unity."

Ava closed her eyes, her thoughts turning inward. The pursuit of authenticity was not just about advocating for change; it was about creating a legacy—a legacy of unity, understanding, and shared purpose.

One day, Ava stood before a holographic projection—a depiction of the citizens of Eudaimonia working together to bring the new vision to life. As she contemplated the transformation that had taken place, a holographic message from Nikos appeared before her. "Ava," his message read, "a balanced society is a reflection of the collective journey toward growth and harmony. Lead with humility and guide citizens toward a future that values authenticity and interconnectedness."

Ava's gaze shifted between the holographic images—the transformation that was visible and the unity that was thriving. A balanced Eudaimonia was not just a goal; it was a reality that demonstrated the power of authenticity and unity to shape a brighter future.

One evening, as Ava sat alone in her apartment, surrounded by holographic displays, a holographic message from Emma appeared before her. "Ava," the message read, "a balanced Eudaimonia is a reflection of your growth and evolution. Allow it to remind you of the transformative power of authenticity in fostering unity and shaping the destiny of a society."

Ava smiled, a profound sense of fulfillment filling her. The holographic displays were no longer just symbols of growth and connection; they were symbols of a balanced Eudaimonia—a society that had embraced its authenticity and was now thriving in unity and harmony.

summary

"Elixir of Eudaimonia":
In the captivating novel "Elixir of Eudaimonia," the reader is transported to a future era marked by astonishing advancements in health and well-being. Within the utopian society of Eudaimonia, every individual enjoys perfect health, boundless happiness, and a harmonious existence. However, beneath the surface of this seemingly idyllic world lies a tale of intrigue, discovery, and a quest for deeper truths.

The story follows the journey of Ava, a young citizen of Eudaimonia, whose curiosity leads her to unravel the carefully constructed facade of her society. Amid holographic displays of unity and prosperity, Ava encounters Emma, a enigmatic figure from the outside world, who introduces her to a realm beyond Eudaimonia's boundaries. Through Emma's guidance, Ava embarks on an exploration that unveils the secrets behind the society's elixir of perfect health and happiness.

As Ava delves deeper into the heart of Eudaimonia's mysteries, she uncovers forbidden knowledge that challenges the very essence of the utopian vision. She discovers that the elixir of health and happiness conceals a hidden price—one that compromises the authenticity of human experience. Her quest for truth ignites a spark of rebellion as she joins forces with like-minded individuals who yearn for a society that values more than just physical well-being.

In the novel's unfolding narrative across 30 chapters, Ava confronts resistance, navigates personal struggles, and initiates conversations that bridge the gap between different factions. Along the way, she formulates a new vision for Eudaimonia—one that celebrates imperfections, honors diversity, and redefines well-being to encompass emotional and societal dimensions.

The climax of the story arrives as Ava's vision gains traction, leading to a transformation of Eudaimonia's core principles. The holographic displays that once projected illusions of harmony now showcase the power of unity, authenticity, and interconnectedness.

"Elixir of Eudaimonia" captivates readers with its exploration of human nature, the consequences of perfection, and the resilience of the human spirit in the face of deception. Through Ava's journey, the novel paints a vivid portrait of a society at the crossroads, challenging readers to consider the true meaning of health, happiness, and the value of embracing the complexity of human existence.

With its compelling characters and thought-provoking themes, "Elixir of Eudaimonia" invites readers to ponder the delicate balance between utopia and reality, and to reflect on the elixirs we seek to enrich our lives.